BIOMATERIALS - PROPERTIES, PRODUCTION AND DEVICES SERIES

BIODEGRADABLE COMPOSITES FOR BONE REGENERATION

BIOMATERIALS - PROPERTIES, PRODUCTION AND DEVICES SERIES

Biomaterials in Blood-Contacting Devices: Complications and Solutions
Meng-Jiy Wang and Wei-Bor Tsai
2010. ISBN: 978-1-60876-784-7

Surface Modification of Titanium for Biomaterial Applications
Kyo-Han Kim, R. Narayanan and Tapash R. Rautray
2010. ISBN: 978-1-60876-539-3

Calcium Orthophosphate-Based Biocomposites and Hybrid Biomaterials
Sergey V. Dorozhkin
2010. ISBN: 978-1-60876-941-4

Biodegradable Composites for Bone Regeneration
Luigi Calandrelli, Paola Laurienzo and Adriana Oliva
2010. ISBN: 978-1-60876-957-5

BIOMATERIALS - PROPERTIES, PRODUCTION AND DEVICES SERIES

BIODEGRADABLE COMPOSITES FOR BONE REGENERATION

LUIGI CALANDRELLI
PAOLA LAURIENZO
AND
ADRIANA OLIVA

Nova Science Publishers, Inc.
New York

Copyright © 2010 by Nova Science Publishers, Inc.

All rights reserved. No part of this book may be reproduced, stored in a retrieval system or transmitted in any form or by any means: electronic, electrostatic, magnetic, tape, mechanical photocopying, recording or otherwise without the written permission of the Publisher.

For permission to use material from this book please contact us:
Telephone 631-231-7269; Fax 631-231-8175
Web Site: http://www.novapublishers.com

NOTICE TO THE READER

The Publisher has taken reasonable care in the preparation of this book, but makes no expressed or implied warranty of any kind and assumes no responsibility for any errors or omissions. No liability is assumed for incidental or consequential damages in connection with or arising out of information contained in this book. The Publisher shall not be liable for any special, consequential, or exemplary damages resulting, in whole or in part, from the readers' use of, or reliance upon, this material.

Independent verification should be sought for any data, advice or recommendations contained in this book. In addition, no responsibility is assumed by the publisher for any injury and/or damage to persons or property arising from any methods, products, instructions, ideas or otherwise contained in this publication.

This publication is designed to provide accurate and authoritative information with regard to the subject matter covered herein. It is sold with the clear understanding that the Publisher is not engaged in rendering legal or any other professional services. If legal or any other expert assistance is required, the services of a competent person should be sought. FROM A DECLARATION OF PARTICIPANTS JOINTLY ADOPTED BY A COMMITTEE OF THE AMERICAN BAR ASSOCIATION AND A COMMITTEE OF PUBLISHERS.

LIBRARY OF CONGRESS CATALOGING-IN-PUBLICATION DATA

Available upon request.
ISBN: 978-1-60876-957-5

Published by Nova Science Publishers, Inc. † New York

Contents

Preface		vii
Abstract		1
Chapter 1	Introduction	3
Chapter 2	Realization and Performance Analysis of PCL/ Silica Nanocomposites for Bone Regeneration	15
Chapter 3	Novel Injectable Alginate/ N-Succinylchitosan/ Calcium Sulphate Composites as Bone-Defects Fillers	39
References		53
Index		65

Preface

In the present book, after briefly summarizing recent literature concerning modification and applications of these materials, several recent developments of bio-composites containing silica nanoparticles or calcium sulphate intended for bone regeneration are reported. The composites are characterized with respect to their chemical-physical and mechanical properties. Their bio-compatibility and capacity to induce the osteoblastic phenotype in human bone marrow mesenchymal stem cells have been assessed. The authors focus on two particular systems based on either natural or synthetic bio-polymers with different biofillers: alginate/chitosan blends with calcium sulphate and poly(-caprolactone) with silica nanoparticles.

ABSTRACT

Osteoinductive materials are strongly searched in reconstructive surgery. Polymer based composites are ideal candidate, as they couple the ease of processing of polymers (by melt or by injection and hardening) with the mechanical reinforcement of fillers, once interfacial adhesion is assured. Moreover, an appropriate choice of the filler may enhance the bone regeneration activity, through cell adhesion or osteoinduction. In this respect hydroxyapatite and calcium sulphate are good candidates. As organic binder, a wide choice of different polymers is possible: biocompatible and biodegradable natural polymers such as polysaccharides and, in more recent years, biocompatible and biodegradable synthetic polyesters are normally employed, with processing methodologies which depend on the intrinsic properties of the polymers (paste injection or injection molding).

In the present chapter, after briefly summarizing recent literature concerning modification and applications of these materials, several recent developments of biocomposites containing silica nanoparticles or calcium sulphate intended for bone regeneration are reported. The composites are characterized with respect to their chemical-physical and mechanical properties. Their biocompatibility and capacity to induce the osteoblastic phenotype in human bone marrow mesenchymal stem cells have been assessed. We will focus on two particular systems based on either natural or synthetic biopolymers with different biofillers: alginate/chitosan blends with calcium sulphate and poly(ε-caprolactone) with silica nanoparticles.

Chapter 1

INTRODUCTION

PRINCIPLES OF TISSUE ENGINEERING

The term "tissue engineering" was defined by the pioneers Langer and Vacanti as "an interdisciplinary field that applies the principles of engineering and life sciences toward the development of biological substitutes that restore, maintain, or improve tissue or organ function" [1]. More recently, MacArthur and Oreffo defined tissue engineering as "understanding the principles of tissue growth, and applying this to produce functional replacement tissue for clinical use" [2].

Tissue engineering can be viewed as the combination of cells, an appropriate scaffold, biologically active molecules and/or suitable mechanical factors, aimed at the replacement, repair, maintenance, and/or improvement of tissue function, thus allowing the advancement of medicine. In effect, "regenerative medicine" is often used as synonymous of "tissue engineering", although the former emphasizes the use of stem cells, rather than already differentiated cells, to produce tissues. Among the numerous regenerative medicine fields, bone tissue engineering is at the forefront of research and clinical applications, representing a great challenge to repair skeletal defects resulting from traumatic injuries, infections, biochemical disorders, tumors and other pathologies.

As afore-mentioned, the main components of a tissue engineered construct are: 1) cells, 2) a scaffold, 3) bioactive factors and/or physical signals.

A polymeric support for tissue growth (also named scaffold) must meet, depending upon the application and together with biocompatibility and biodegradability, several other requirements, as high porous structure, interconnected pore network, and good mechanical strength and flexibility. An example of the structure of a polymer based scaffold (namely poly(lactic acid), PLA), as it appears by scanning electron microscopy (SEM), is reported in Figure 1 (a and b). The dimension of the pores must be comprised between 100 and 300 µm, to allow the cell to penetrate and grow inside the scaffold; furthermore, a high pore interconnectivity is a strict requirement in order to get the formation of new tissue. Figure 1b clearly shows such pore interconnection.

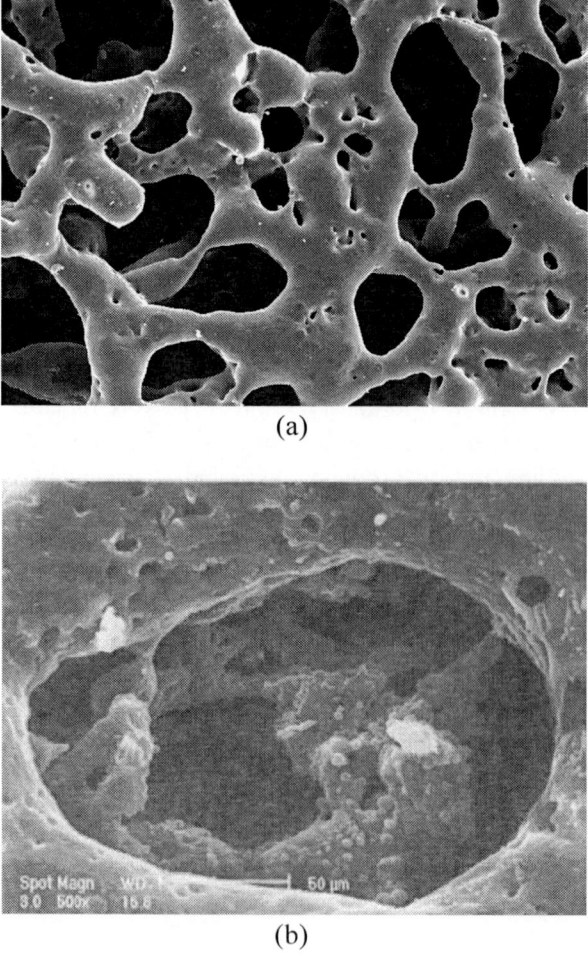

(a)

(b)

Figure 1. (a and b). SEM micrograph of a typical poly(lactic acid) scaffold. A detail of the pore network structure is reported in figure b.

As regards the cellular component, it can consist of either differentiated cells from the tissue of interest or stem cells/precursor cells, but bone tissue engineering using bone marrow stem cells appears the most promising technique for reconstructing bone defects.

Bone marrow is a complex cellular array of stem cells of both hematopoietic and nonhematopoietic lineages. In 1987 Friedenstein et al showed that a specific set of cells (colony forming unit fibroblasts, CFU-F) present in bone marrow can differentiate into different cell types, including osteoblasts [3]. These cells, referred to as mesenchymal stem cells or marrow stromal cells (MSCs), have a great capacity of self-renewal and multipotency. These cells, indeed, can give rise to precursors for bone, cartilage, adipose tissue, tendon, muscle, and marrow stroma [4,5]. In addition, MSCs have been demonstrated to be capable to differentiate into cardiomyocytes, astrocytes and neurons [6-8]. A number of studies on MSCs have demonstrated the great plasticity of these cells and that their fate strictly depends on various environmental signals [9,10].

An ideal bone tissue engineering strategy implies the use of autologous bone marrow MSCs, even if their demonstrated immunoregulatory activity might allow also the use of allogeneic cells [11].

The typical bone tissue regeneration strategy involves either the isolation and ex vivo expansion of cell population within the engineered construct in a bioreactor, followed by implantation, or in situ recruitment of endogenous cells to the implantation site through the use of osteoconductive scaffolds possibly delivering bioactive molecules, such as osteoinductive growth factors ("smart" scaffolds).

A serious drawback to the former approach is represented by the low number of MSCs in bone marrow. In this respect, the utilization of own platelet-rich plasma, that is a rich source of a number of growth factors essential in the modulation of the wound-healing process, can be a method for the rapid ex vivo expansion of MSCs before their clinical application, avoiding the use of heterologous human- or animal-derived growth supplements as well as expensive recombinant growth factors [12].

While in a great number of animal studies the feasibility of bone formation has been reported, in human bone tissue engineering has not always been a clinical success. Among the factors preventing the reaching of a successful outcome, lack of sufficient vascular supply is thought to be the main cause of failure since the vascularization is a key factor in bone tissue engineering [13].

Even if MSCs themselves secrete a large number of bioactive factors capable of creating a regenerative microenvironment at the injury site, which Caplan defines as "trophic activity" [14], and are able to promote the neovascularization through the release of angiogenic factors, it could be necessary, particularly for large bone defects, to stimulate vessel growth and thus improve the oxygen and nutrients supply by adding angiogenetic growth factors, or even endothelial cells, to the tissue engineered construct [13,15].

BIOCOMPATIBILITY TESTING OF MEDICAL DEVICES: "TESTS FOR IN VITRO CYTOTOXICITY (EN ISO 10993-5)"

Upstream to clinical applications in humans, all materials designed for biomedical devices must be submitted to *in vitro* and *in vivo* tests to verify biocompatibility, response and behavior of the interacting cells according to the rules of EN ISO 10993. The standard EN ISO 10993-5, that has been just revised substituting the previous edition 10-years old, contains methods designed to assess the in vitro cytotoxicity of medical devices, namely the biological response of mammalian cells using appropriate biological parameters.

Indeed, ISO 10993-5:2009 describes test methods that specify the incubation of cultured cells in contact with a device and/or extracts of a device either directly or through diffusion. One of these methods, the so-called indirect test (or elution test), represents the first step of the biocompatibility analysis and is widely used and applicable to every type of medical devices. In this method, culture medium containing extractables derived from the tested material, obtained under standard conditions, is applied to a cell layer. The cultures are then returned to the 37°C incubator and periodically examined by microscope for as long as three days. During incubation, any leachable chemicals from the test material can directly interact with the cell layer and induce or not signs of toxicity.

Once proved the absence of cytotoxicity by means of the elution method, materials projected for bone tissue regeneration devices should be subjected to the another *in vitro* approach, that is a direct contact method. In this approach, cell populations typical of the implant site, as well as their progenitors, are cultured directly onto the material under investigation and observed, for a period of days or weeks, in terms of morphological and functional features.

PRINCIPLES OF SYNTHETIC BONE SUBSTITUTES

Bone is a complex and a highly specialized form of connective tissue pertaining to the formation of the skeleton of the body. Bone not only provides mechanical support but also serves as a reservoir for minerals, particularly calcium and phosphate. It is a good example of a dynamic tissue, since it has a unique capability of self-regenerating or self-remodeling to a certain extent throughout the life without leaving a scar [16]. However, many circumstances call for bone grafting owing to bone defects either from traumatic or from non-traumatic destruction. There are multiple methods available for the treatment of bone defects, which includes the traditional methods of autografting and allografting

Although autografting and allografting are clinically considered as good therapies, they have limitations. For example, supply of autograft is limited and there is a possibility of pathogen transfer from allograft. Accordingly, there is a great need for the use of synthetic bone grafts. Nowadays, numerous synthetic bone graft materials, both single- and multi-phases, are available which are capable of alleviating some of the practical complications associated with the autogenous or allogeneic bones.

Several classes of materials such as ceramics, metals and polymers have been used as artificial bone to fill bone cavities and to refill bony structures [17,18]. In most of the cases, metals and ceramics are used in hard tissue applications, whilst polymers in soft tissue applications due to their mechanical properties. Although there is good progress in bone grafting using synthetic bone grafts, the way in which they execute their functions *in vivo* is quite different and most of them differ from natural bone either compositionally or structurally. Further, a single-phase material (also called monolithic) does not always provide all the essential features required for bone growth, which leads to incessant investigation in search of an ideal bone graft. There is, therefore, a great need for engineered multi-phase materials (also called composites) with structure and composition similar to natural bone [19].Composites are widely used in both soft and hard tissue applications.

Being the mineral phase of bone mainly composed by natural hydroxyapatite (HA), cements based on synthetic HA are among the most investigated materials for dental and orthopedic applications in reconstructive surgery. HA is employed as substitute for defective bones because of its biocompatibility, bone bonding ability, osteoconductivity, non-toxic and non-inflammatory effects [20-26]. Nevertheless, HA cements are hard (not injectable and mouldable) [27,28], brittle, and not suitable for handling and processing [28-31]. Consequently, several composite and nanocomposite materials based on natural or synthetic biodegradable polymers with HA or its precursors (i.e., calcium phosphates) have been proposed and tested [32-38]. Biocomposite implantation materials based on calcium phosphates substantially expanded the possibility of restorative and substitutive osteoplastic surgery, mainly in dentistry, maxillofacial surgery, and neurosurgery.

The term nanocomposite can be defined as a heterogeneous combination of two or more materials in which at least one of those materials is on a nanometer-scale. Natural bone itself is a true nanocomposite composed mainly of HA nanocrystallites in the collagen-rich organic matrix [39,40]; thereby choosing a HA/collagen nanocomposite as a bone graft material is an added advantage [41], as it mimics the bone components [42]. Nanocrystalline HA promotes osteoblast cells adhesion, differentiation, and proliferation, osteointegration and deposition of calcium containing minerals on its surface better than microcrystalline HA, thus enhancing the formation of new bone tissue within a short period [43-45]. Nanocomposites have been largely studied mainly for their superior mechanical characteristics; nevertheless, more recent studies are aimed at giving and using bioactivity and osteoconductivity. The main role of osteoconductive grafts is to serve as a structural framework through which the host bone cells infiltrate and regenerate a new bone tissue. Many researchers have attempted to give osteoconductivity to bone cement based on natural or synthetic biopolymers by introducing different bioactive fillers. Biological and clinical testing made it possible to establish that the biological activity of materials and their compatibility with an organism are primarily related to the presence in their composition of HA and tricalcium phosphate (β-TCP); more recently, ceramic fillers as silica nanoparticles [46-48] or different salts, as calcium sulphate [49-50], have been proposed. However, the interfacial strength between bioactive filler and the organic polymer is of concern because of the lack of adhesion between the two phases, resulting in an early failure at the interface. In addition, the distribution of the nanometric filler in the polymeric matrix must be homogeneous, in order to increase its surface exposure. These parameters are fundamental to induce the osteoconducting ability of the biocomposite.

Nanocomposites can be made, conventionally, by blending a heterogeneous combination of two or more materials, differing in morphology or composition. It is well known that blending of multiple materials with different characteristics leads to composites with tailor-made properties, but it is quite difficult to control homogeneity and uniformity of the reinforcing phases. The crystallites are not uniform in size, and are often aggregated and randomly distributed into the matrix; therefore there is no structural uniformity observed that is close to natural bone. Further, there is no sign of chemical interaction between mineral and organic phases, which is probably due to the lack of suitable interfacial-bonding. So, it is clear that the first research effort must consist in optimizing nanocomposite processing conditions and interfacial characteristics. Therefore, if nanometer-sized bioactive ceramics can be dispersed homogeneously and bonded covalently to the polymer phase at the molecular level, all problems are likely to be solved. The improvement of the adhesion between the ceramic fillers and the biopolymer could be achieved using a coupling agent; surface modification of the inorganic particles by organic molecules also is an effective means to manipulate the inter-surface properties, and develop optimized biomaterials [51]. A brief overview of the most promising polymers and inorganic fillers used to realize biocomposites for bone tissue engineering, together with the chemical strategies developed for the optimization of their properties, is hereafter reported.

POLYMERS FOR BONE TISSUE ENGINEERING

Biodegradable natural and synthetic polymers as well as some non-biodegradable polymers, which are currently used for cartilage tissue engineering, have been described as organic components in materials and composites for bone regeneration [52,53]. Polymers have distinct advantages over the ceramic materials. Bioactive ceramics have chemical composition resembling that of natural bone but they are inherently brittle and have low biodegradation rates, which limit their clinical uses [54]. On the other hand, the mechanical properties and biodegradation rate of polymers can be tailored to a certain extent for specific applications. Re-absorbable or degradable biomaterials containing the high MW hyaluronic acid have been extensively explored for tissue engineering applications. Biomaterials based on hyaluronic acid, with excellent histocompatibility and biodegradability, were prepared for the synthetic bio-skin and biosynthetic osteo-cartilage used for the reconstruction of tissues. The addition of growth factors and cytokines promoted cell migration, proliferation and formation of a new tissue [55]. Also natural polyesters based on hydroxyvalerate were tested for repair of the musculoskeletal tissues. In vivo experiments indicated that, for some compositions, they may perhaps be the most suitable polymeric material for this application [56].

Advanced tissue engineering involves the use of 3D polymeric scaffolds implanted at the defective site. They provide frameworks for cells to attach, proliferate, and form extracellular matrix (ECM). Biodegradable scaffolds should be bioabsorbed at a predetermined rate and the space initially occupied by them should be fully replaced by the regenerated tissue [57]. Several methods are used to produce scaffolds from both natural and synthetic polymers; among them, the electrospinning technique allows the preparation of scaffolds from uniform nanofibers with mean diameter of 260 nm, that closely mimic the native ECM found in the human body and are expected to support active tissue regeneration. Scaffolds suitable for bone tissue engineering were prepared by combining ceramic materials with biocompatible, water soluble polymers based on N-vinylpyrrolidone and acrolein diethyl acetal [58]. Synthetic biodegradable polyesters, as poly(L-lactide) (PLLA), poly(D,L-lactide-co-glycolide) (PLGA), polycaprolactone (PCL) and their copolymers or combinations of them have been often used for the preparation of porous scaffolds. However, the hydrophobicity, the acidity of their decomposition products, and the self acceleration of their degradation, have constituted serious drawbacks. Hybrid materials based on synthetic polymers and collagen, the main organic constituent of the human bone [59], have been proposed. In vivo studies showed that a hybrid scaffold has a high degree of tissue compatibility. Calcium deposition appeared 4 weeks after insertion [58]. PLLA/collagen scaffolds seemed to be preferable to pure collagen sponge as maintained the original shape throughout the implantation period of 8 weeks, while the collagen sponge collapsed [60]. Development of bone analogues on a biomimetic PCL/ceramic polymer was explored. Human marrow stem cells were able to adhere, migrate, and differentiate on these biodegradable scaffolds, which degraded much faster than PCL alone [61].

The usually low manufacture costs related to their large agricultural availability and renewability are additional advantages of natural biopolymers. Furthermore, their versatility of chemical structures and their well-known chemistry allow the development of advanced functionalized materials that can match several varied requirements [62-64]. Among the biopolymers, polysaccharides have the widest medical applications due to their nontoxicity, water solubility, or high swelling ability induced by simple modification, stability to pH variation, and a broad variety of chemical structures [65,66]. In particular, natural polysaccharides are widely employed in bone regeneration techniques, in order to overcome drawbacks of mineral bone graft substitutes, such as hydroxyapatite and calcium sulphate.

Special attention has been given recently to chitosan and its derivatives, in combination with HA and various natural and synthetic polymers. Grafted chitosans are extensively investigated for applications in cell transplantation and for tissue regeneration [67-69]. Chitosan has been shown to improve wound healing [70-72] and enhance bone formation [71-74]. In addition, it is non-toxic, bioresorbable and non-immunogenic [75-77]. For these reasons, it has been suggested to possess biological properties suitable for clinical applications. Chitosan scaffolds for bone tissue engineering have been widely investigated [78-80] and showed to enhance bone formation both in vitro and in vivo [81]. In addition, chitosan has excellent filmogenic properties, and its biodegradation kinetics is slower than that showed by other biocompatible polymers (i.e. collagen) [82]. Feng Zhao et al. [36] prepared a biodegradable HA/chitosan-gelatine network composite as a three dimensional biomimetic scaffold for bone tissue engineering. Besides, an interesting case was reported by Murugan et al. [83] who prepared a bioresorbable composite bone paste based on HA in conjugation with chitosan for bone repair and regeneration. They used a wet chemical method at low temperature and obtained a HA composite with a decreased bioresorption and particle migration rate with respect to HA bioceramics.

Biocomposite nano-scaffolds of chitosan/poly(vinylalcohol)/HA prepared by electrospinning showed a well interconnected pore network structure with nanofibrous morphology and were considered as a promising material for bone tissue regeneration [84]. However, several efforts have been devoted to functionalize chitosan, because of its poor workability and scarce water solubility at neutral pH [85,86].

Great interest in biomedical field has been given also to alginate. Alginate is a safe, biocompatible natural polysaccharide obtained from marine algae used in food and biomedical applications, mainly for its capacity to crosslink in presence of bivalent ions under very mild conditions [87-89]. Alginate/HA and alginate/collagen/HA composites have been proposed as scaffold materials for bone tissue engineering [90]. Parhi et al developed an alginate-hydroxyapatite biocomposite, in which the mineral phase was nucleated on alginate chains by precipitation method to obtain a biomimetic artificial bonelike composite [91]. A polymeric composite made up of nanohydroxyapatite and alginate was formed as a result of in situ nucleation of hydroxyapatite on alginate polymeric chain [92].

SILICA-BASED MATERIALS AND NANOPARTICLES FOR BONE REGENERATION

Silica, the mineral of which sand is made, is generally inert in the body and can be modified easily using a variety of well-established chemical reactions. As such, researchers have considered silica an ideal candidate material from which to create multifunctional nanoparticles. Silica nanoparticles (SNP) have been widely used for biosensing and catalytic applications due to their large surface area to volume ratio, straightforward manufacture and the possibility to be doped and/or functionalized with fluorescent molecules [93,94], magnetic nanoparticles [95] or semiconducting nanocrystals [96]. Porous silica nanoparticles hold promise as drug delivery vehicles, imaging agents, and even nanoscale collection devices for cancer markers [97]. SNP can be prepared using several techniques, including the widely used Stobër technique and the water-in-oil nanoemulsion system. The former is based on the simple hydrolysis of a silica precursor in alcoholic medium in the presence of ammonia; the latter uses water droplets inside of reverse micelles as nanoreactors. The size of the final nanospheres is mainly regulated by the dimension of the water droplets and, therefore, by the molar ratio of water to surfactant and by the molar ratio of water to the precursor. Other relevant parameters are the molar ratio of the precursor to the catalyst, the reactivity of the precursor, the total time and temperature of the reaction. As previously said, silica based nanoparticles find their use particularly in bioanalysis if these are conjugated to recognize biocomponents. In the conjugation process, special elements that interact with the analyses are carefully selected. Using various methods these elements can suitably attached to the silica nanoparticle surface. There are several biochemical binding approaches for modifying the silica nanoparticle surfaces to contain functional groups. These functional groups are useful for further modification in surface and biomolecule immobilization. So far the research has been successfully completed on biochemical groups including amines, carboxyls, thiols, however various other molecules including oligonucleotides, enzymes and other proteins are being used for immobilizing onto the nanoparticles. Application of such organically modified silica nanoparticles as a nonviral vector for efficient *in vivo* gene delivery has been reported, where highly monodispersed, stable aqueous suspension of nanoparticles were surface-functionalized with amino groups for binding of DNA [98].

For what concerns applications of silica nanoparticles in bone tissue regeneration, several examples of nanocomposites based on acrylic matrices containing silica nanoparticles as bioactive filler for bone cement [46,99] and resin for dental applications [100,101] have been reported. The authors always observed high mechanical properties in addition to crystalline apatite formation on implants in simulated body fluid (SBF), proving that silica nanoparticles act as a nucleation site for several salts, as calcium phosphates, that promote formation of HA in *in vivo* simulating conditions. Formation of an apatite layer and favourable mechanical properties were also observed on PCL/silica nanocomposites [47,102,103].

To improve the interface with the organic matrix, silica based nanoparticles can be chemically or physically modified [104]. Different non-covalent mechanisms, as hydrophobic interactions [105-107], ionic interactions [108,109], and π-π interactions [110-112], are involved in the physical adsorption of functional molecules onto the surface of nanoparticles. The silanization method is widely used for chemical modification; as a conventional silanization reagent, trimethoxysilylpropyl–diethylenetriamine (DETA) has been reported to introduce amine groups onto the surfaces of silica nanoparticles [113]. Similarly, trimethoxysilane–PEG and trifluoroethylester PEG silane have been shown to link to silica based nanospheres and introduce PEG molecules onto the nanosphere surface [104,114-116]. Vinyl modified silica nanoparticles have been photopolymerized with acrylic monomers to develop polymethacrylate-silica hybrid/nanocomposite dental materials characterized by low volume shrinkage [117].

Nowadays, along with the use of nanoparticles, several examples can be found in literature concerning multi-phase materials intended for bone regeneration based on silica. Non-woven silica gel fabric prepared by the electrospinning method provided a suitable morphological architecture for the differentiation of pre-osteoblastic cells and osteoconductivity [118]. Nano-silica-fused whiskers combined with calcium phosphate cements (CPC) were used as fillers in a resin matrix-based composite. The role of nano-silica was fundamentally to reinforce the CPC-based composites. The mechanical properties of the CPC/silica-whisker composites nearly matched those of cortical bone and trabecular bone [119]. As the general drawback of biocomposite based on HA and β-TCP consists in a substantial decrease in the activity of calcium phosphates in a physiological medium, since their synthesis requires a high temperature (above 1200°C), biocomposite synthesized by sintering HA and β-TCP powders and an amorphous silicate matrix at temperatures below 800°C makes possible to preserve the defects of the HA structure in the material and, accordingly, its relatively high resorption capacity. Further, the main advantages of such implant materials are their mechanical strength, which is comparable to that of bone tissue, and their suitability for the production of structural implants. At the same time, the related porous biocomposites in their physicomechanical parameters are at the same level as spongy bone tissues [120].

THE USE OF CALCIUM SULPHATE IN BONE REGENERATION

The hemihydrate form of calcium sulphate ($CaSO_4 \cdot \frac{1}{2} H_2O$, CHS), better known as Plaster of Paris, is one of the calcium salts most investigated as a substitute for bone graft [49,50]. It has been demonstrated that it can prevent the growth of soft connective tissue in the cavity and that it also has osteoconductive properties [121]. It is in fact reported that gypsum, in contact with body fluids, forms calcium phosphate deposits which are finally responsible for conducting and accelerating bone formation [122-124]. Addition of water to CHS powder elicits an exothermic reaction with the end product being the dihydrate form of calcium sulphate ($CaSO_4 \cdot 2H_2O$, gypsum). The as obtained product is a paste with good handling properties and mouldability which in several minutes gets a hard cement. Despite its efficiency, the potential applications are limited by its rapid *in vivo* resorption and its brittleness [125]. Novel calcium sulphate/polymer systems in which CHS can be encapsulated in a polymeric biodegradable and biocompatible matrix, in order to retain the structural integrity and decrease the bioresorption rate, have been recently developed [126,127]. In one case, poly(ε-caprolactone) (PCL), a biodegradable and non-cytotoxic polyester [30,32,128], currently regarded as a soft and hard-tissue compatible material including resorbable sutures, drug delivery system and, recently, bone graft substitutes [30,128,129], has been used to realize these networks. In the other case, encapsulation of calcium sulphate in hydrogels based on blends of natural, biocompatible polysaccharides got a hard cement, characterized by good mechanical properties and slower resorption rate.

In this chapter, some novel composite materials for bone tissue regeneration based on biodegradable polymers are described. We pointed on two different systems.

The first system we dealt with is a PCL-based composite with silica nanoparticles. The nanoparticles have been chemically modified on their surface with PCL of reduced molecular weight to improve interface adhesion with the polymer matrix; successive introduction of vinyl groups allowed grafting onto PCL. The resulting nanocomposite is characterized by improved mechanical and osteoconductive properties.

The second one consists of a blend of natural polysaccharides, chitosan and alginate, entrapping calcium sulphate as osteoinducting phase. We showed how it was possible to obtain a material of superior characteristics, due to a synergistic effect between the two polymers at a given composition of the blend.

Chapter 2

REALIZATION AND PERFORMANCE ANALYSIS OF PCL/ SILICA NANOCOMPOSITES FOR BONE REGENERATION

Luigi Calandrelli, Fulvio Della Ragione, Mario Malinconico, Adriana Oliva

Nanocomposites of PCL and silica, in which the silica nanoparticles have been modified to provide a chemical graft onto PCL and so improve interfacial adhesion, are hereafter described.

The nanoparticles were prepared following the Stöber method [130], as described in the Experimental (see below), and then characterized by Transmission Electron Microscopy (TEM) (figure 2). From the morphological analysis we desume that the so obtained nanoparticles are spherical in shape with dimensions comprised between 100 and 200 nm.

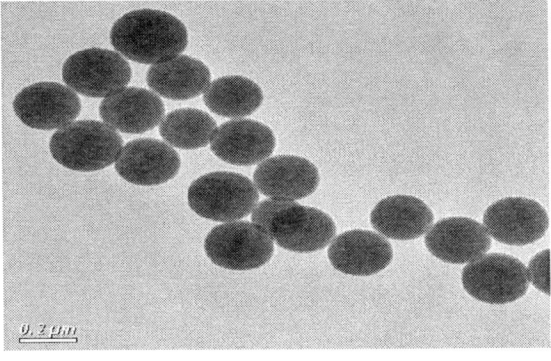

Figure 2. TEM micrograph of Aerosil® 90 silica nanoparticles.

MECHANICAL ALLOYS
(CHEMICAL PHYSICAL AND MECHANICAL PROPERTIES)

Before the realization of the functionalised nanocomposites, mechanical alloys, i.e., nanocomposites obtained simply by mixing unmodified PCL and unmodified silica nanoparticles, A90 (see Experimental), in matrix PCL with a percentage of silica of 1, 3 and 5% have been prepared and characterized. The scope of this preliminary study was to verify if in the absence of specific interfacial interactions, but simply with the addition of a nanometric filler to the polymer matrix, the physical and mechanical chemical properties of the PCL could improve. As it is shown from Table 1, the calorimetric analysis (DSC) of the PCL evidences the temperatures of fusion (T_f) and of onset and endset of fusion (Tonset and Tendset), the degree of crystallinity in heating (Xc^1) and cooling (Xc^2) and the temperatures of crystallization (Tc), glass transition (Tg) and degradation (Td). The presence of the nanosilica has not caused any variation of the transition temperatures (T of fusion, T of crystallization and T of glass transition). Also the thermal stability of composites did not seem to be influenced from the presence of the silica.

The tensile tests carried out in order to estimate parameters such as stress at break, Young's modulus and extensibility, indicate that increasing the percentage of silica leads to a corresponding increase of the modulus and a diminution of the extensibility (Table 2). This to demonstrate that it is possible to increase the structural properties of the PCL without depressing in considerable measure the plastic properties of the material. (Note: Table 2 is broken)

Table 1. Thermal parameters of PCL

PCL	T_f (°C)*	Xc^1	Tc (°C)	Xc^2	Tg (°C)	Td (°C)
	58 (52-65)	42	32	38	-60	383

* in parentheses, the T of onset and end of fusion are reported.

Table 2. Mechanical parameters of plain PCL and of PCL/A90 silica nanocomposites

PCL/A90	Stress at break (MPa) (± 15%)	Young's Modulus (MPa) (± 4%)	Elongation at break (%) (± 15%)
100/0	44	380	1500
99/1 (1%)	40	430	1366
97/3 (3%)	37	500	1400
95/5 (5%)	37	520	1300

CHEMICAL MODIFICATION AND CHARACTERIZATION OF NANOCOMPOSITES

It is found in literature that in presence of specific interfacial interactions between matrix and nano-reinforcement, it is possible to exalt the performances of the nanocomposites. In order to improve the interfacial adhesion between the matrix and the nanoparticles, to promote the formation of a reactive interphase and to increase the hydrophylicity, opportune chemical modifications have been carried out either on the polyester chain or on the surface of the nanoparticles. In particular, the PCL has been functionalised introducing in chain approximately 10% by weight of glycidilmethacrylate (GMA) with the help of dibenzoylperoxide (DBPO). Nanoparticles of silica, characterized from the presence on the surface of vinyl groups (Aerosil® R7200), hence in a position to link them to the GMA through the creation of a covalent bond during the GMA radical homopolymerization, has been therefore added in the Rheocord and the mixing was continued to 100°C for further 10 min. In figure 3 we show the sequence of the reactions that leads to the formation of the functionalised nanocomposites.

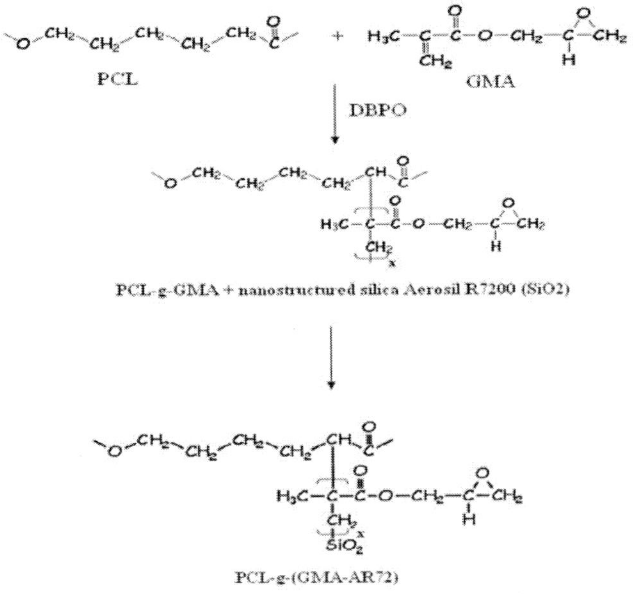

Figure 3. The sequence of reactions which lead to the formation of functionalised nanocomposites. (Note: caption should be at bottom of page 17)

The functionalised nanocomposites (containing 1, 3 or 5% of nanoparticles, as well as previously described mechanical alloys) do not have demonstrated substantial and meaningful differences to the thermal analysis compared to results obtained for mechanical alloys. On the systems so prepared, mechanical tests at low and high deformation speed have been carried out. In Table 3 the results of the tensile tests are reported. As it is possible to observe, the presence of the nanoparticles of silica generates an increment of the Young's modulus. In turn, such increment results to be more meaningful once the chemical modifications so far illustrated are introduced (see Table 2 for a comparison). In this last case, the variations recorded are in accordance with the content of nanoreinforcement that acts hence as stress concentrator, hardening the system.

Table 3. Mechanical parameters of plain PCL and of PCL-g-(GMA-AR72) functionalised silica nanocomposites

Sample (silica %)	Stress at break (MPa) (±15%)	Young's Modulus (MPa) (± 4%)	Elongation at break (%) (±15%)
PCL	44	380	1500
PCL-g-(GMA-AR72) 1%	24	509	563
PCL-g-(GMA-AR72) 3%	19	566	443
PCL-g-(GMA-AR72) 5%	20	563	510
PCL-g-GMA/A90 1%	22	517	577
PCL/A90 1%	40	430	1366

Moreover, we notice from Table 3 that the increment of the Young's modulus, although significant when increasing the percentage of nanosilica, turns out to be nearly equal in the percentage of the 3 and 5% thus demonstrating that the increase of the total surface of the nanoparticles determines the impossibility for the polymer matrix to coat it all. As a consequence, high percentages of nanosilica caused the birth of structural defects with worsening of the mechanical properties or at least an invariance of properties. Moreover, tensile tests have been carried out also on the nanocomposite in which the functionalisation regards only PCL (PCL-g-GMA/A90 1%) and on the corresponding mechanical alloy (PCL/A90 1%). In the direct comparison we notice that the single chemical modification of the PCL phase itself determines an increment of the mechanical properties that approach those of the functionalised nanocomposite, while the mechanical alloy has slightly better properties compared to neat PCL but clearly inferior to those of the PCL-g-GMA/A90 1% composite.

MORPHOLOGIC ANALYSIS (SEM)

Fracture surfaces of mechanical as well as functionalised systems have been observed to the Scanning Electron Microscope (SEM). Nanocomposites between not functionalised PCL and not functionalised silica (mechanical alloys PCL/A90 1%, PCL/A90 3%, PCL/A90 5%, (Figure 4), show, at least till 3%, a good dispersion of the nanofillers in the polymer matrix, but an insufficient interfacial adhesion is found. At 5% begins to evidence aggregations of the nanofillers. The alloy prepared with the functionalised PCL and the not functionalised silica (PCL-g-GMA/A90 1%) shows a morphology significantly different from the analogous mechanical alloy (PCL/A90 1%) (Figure 5) characterized by an elevated interconnection between the phases evidenced from the extensive covering of the nanofillers with the polymer matrix. In Figure 5b the interconnection is better appreciated. These phenomena boast in the nanocomposites where both the components are functionalised (PCL-g-(GMA-AR72) 1%, PCL-g-(GMA-AR72) 3%, PCL-g-(GMA-AR72) 5%; Figure 6). In fact in the composite at 1% a greater adhesion of the nanofiller to the polymer matrix is observed. The phenomenon then becomes evident in the composite with 3% of functionalised silica and seems to become stabilized, without great changes, in that with 5% of functionalised silica. It is interesting to emphasize that, as a result of this covering of the nanofillers with the matrix, for the same composition the surface of the functionalised system seems much more covered from nanofillers than the analogous alloy not made compatible.

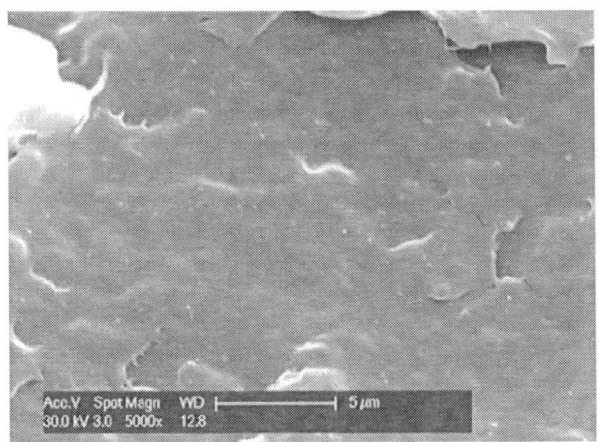

(a) (Note: (a) at bottom of page 19)

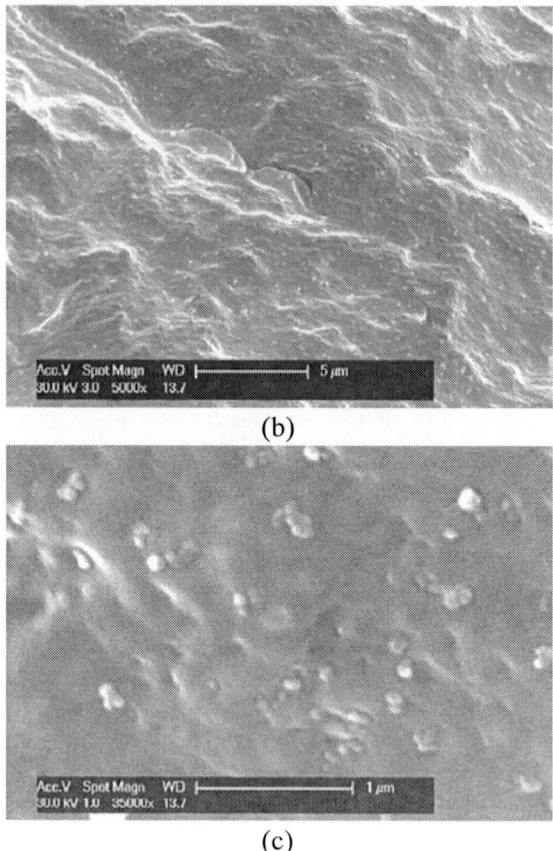

Figure 4. SEM micrographs of: (a) PCL/A90 1%, (b) PCL/A90 3%, (c) PCL/A90 5% nanocomposites.

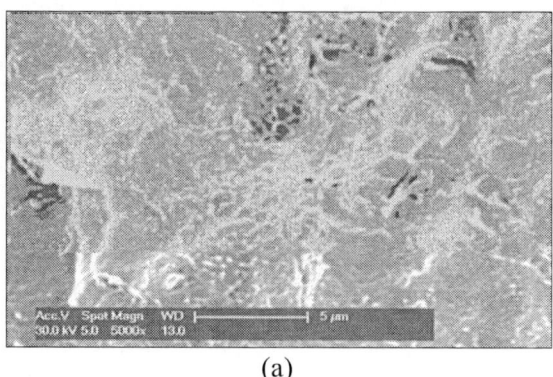

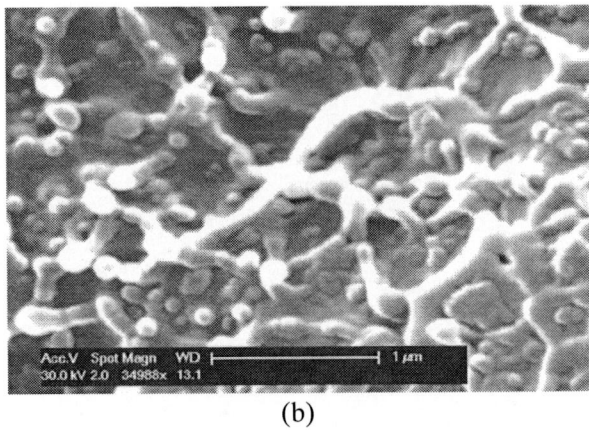

(b)

Figure 5. SEM micrographs of PCL-g-GMA/A90 1% at different magnifications.

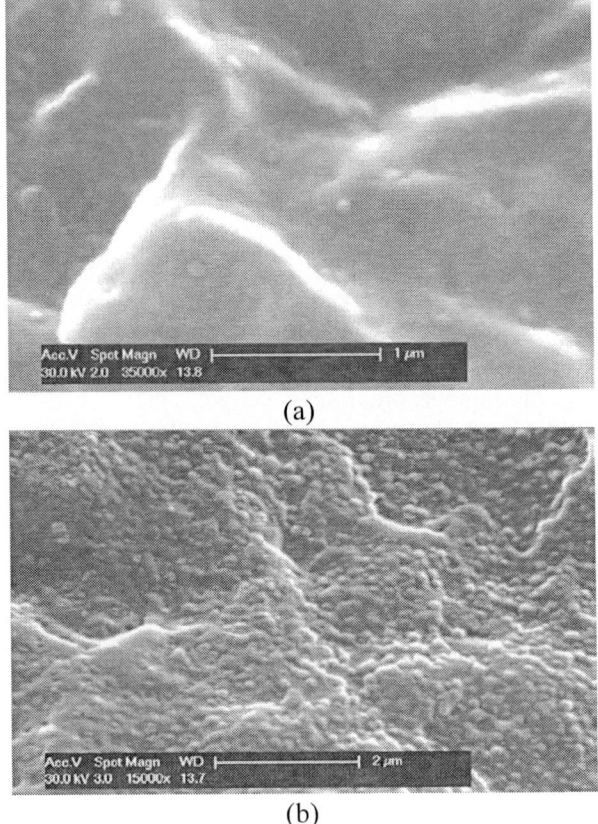

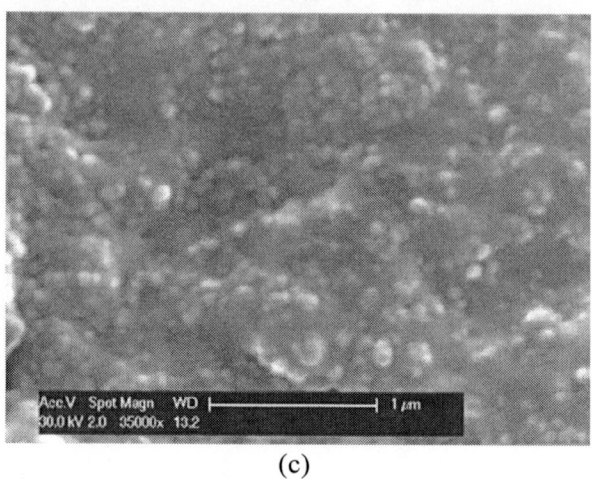
(c)

Figure 6. SEM micrographs of : (a) (PCL-g-(GMA-AR72) 1%, (b) PCL-g-(GMA-AR72) 3%, (c) PCL-g-(GMA-AR72) 5%.

As above mentioned, the functionalisation of the PCL with glicydilmethacrylate (GMA) was required to improve the hydrophilicity of the employed PCL. On the basis of preliminary biological results (see next paragraph), it appeared that the epoxy function could be responsible for the decreased adhesion of cells compared to PCL. GMA has been therefore replaced with butylmethacrylate (BMA). BMA is to be considered a monofunctional monomer as the only reactive group is the double bond, while GMA is a bifunctional acrylic with two reactive groups, namely the double bond and the epoxy group. In Figure 7 we show the reactions that lead to the functionalisation of the PCL with the BMA and the nanostructured silica. The preparation of the nanocomposites is the same as previously shown.

As for the previously described system, nanocomposites with a percentage of 3% by weight were prepared and compared to pure PCL and pure PCL-g-BMA. As for PCL-g-GMA, also (Note: delete "PCL") PCL-g-BMA was purified by dissolution in chloroform and precipitation in cyclohexane to get read of the unreacted monomers.

On the prepared nanocomposites mechanical tensile tests are performed as previously described, in view of getting a comprehensive comparison of the properties with those collected on nanocomposites based on PCL-g-GMA, i.e. PCL-g-(GMA-AR72).

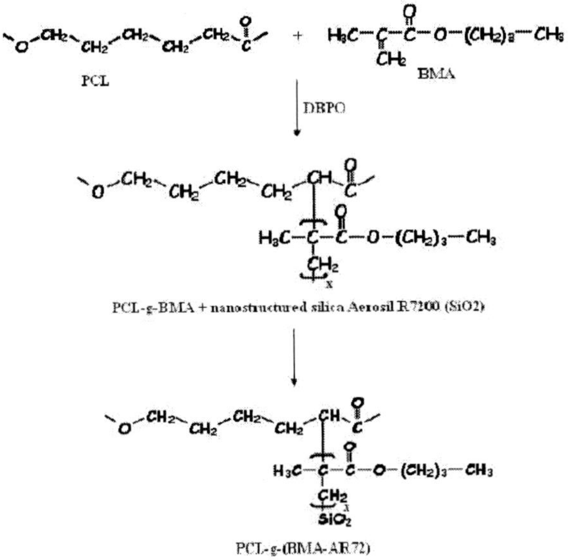

Figura 7. Preparation of PCL-g-(BMA-AR72) nanocomposite.

Table 4. Comparison of mechanical parameters of PCL-g-GMA, PCL-g-BMA, and their functionalized silica nanocomposites (Note: broken Table)

Sample	Stress at break (MPa) (± 15%)	Young's Modulus (MPa) (± 4%)	Elongation at break (%) (± 15%)
PCL-g-GMA	23	510	567
PCL-g-(GMA-AR72) 3%	19	566	443
PCL-g-BMA	21	520	559
PCL-g-(BMA-AR72) 3%	22	560	479

The results shown in Table 4 evidence an increase in Young modulus of the nanocomposite with respect to functionalized PCL, but the values are so close to each other that we can state no big difference in physical properties occurs when GMA group is replaced by BMA.

BIOLOGICAL EVALUATION

ISO 10993-5:2009 standards describe test methods that specify the incubation of cultured cells in contact with a device (direct contact test) and/or extracts of a device (elution test). In the direct contact method, the cells were cultured directly on the material under investigation and observed, for a period of days or weeks, in terms of morphological and functional features. Although the limits of all in vitro studies, including the present, are related to the impossibility of reproducing the complex of the biological events that happen in vivo, nevertheless this type of approach can allow to investigate in detail the interaction between cells and implant surface. This initial phase is crucial, being the contact of cells with the biomaterial the basis for all the following events, including the expression of biochemical specific markers, as well as the deposition of an organized extracellular matrix and its mineralization.

We investigated *in vitro* the biocompatibility of the novel biocomposites as well as their capacity to induce the osteogenic differentiation of human bone marrow stromal cells. Cell proliferation and osteogenic differentiation were evaluated by MTT assay, alkaline phosphatase (AP) activity, osteocalcin (OC) content measurement.

Upstream to the *in vitro* studies with human cells, we analyzed the biocompatibility of the unmodified nanocomposite (PCL/A90) with different amount of silica nanoparticles (1, 3, and 5%) performing a set of elution tests in which murine cells (NIH-3T3) were subjected for 24 and 48 h to both 100% and 50% extracts of these materials (Figures 8A and 8B, respectively). A certain toxicity at increasing percentages of silica was evident mostly with 100% extracts.

On the basis of this result and of the mechanical features of the PCL/A90 3% nanocomposite, which resembled the characteristics of bone tissue more than the others, we selected this composition as the starting material for the functionalised nanocomposites.

The following list reports all the materials tested on bone marrow stromal cells in a direct contact method:

- PCL
- PCL/A90 (not functionalized nanocomposite)
- PCL-g-GMA (functionalized PCL)
- PCL-g-GMA/A90 (functionalized PCL + nanosilica)
- PCL-g-(GMA-AR72) (functionalized PCL + functionalized nanosilica)
- PCL-g-BMA (functionalized PCL)
- PCL-g-(BMA-AR72) (functionalized PCL + functionalized nanosilica)

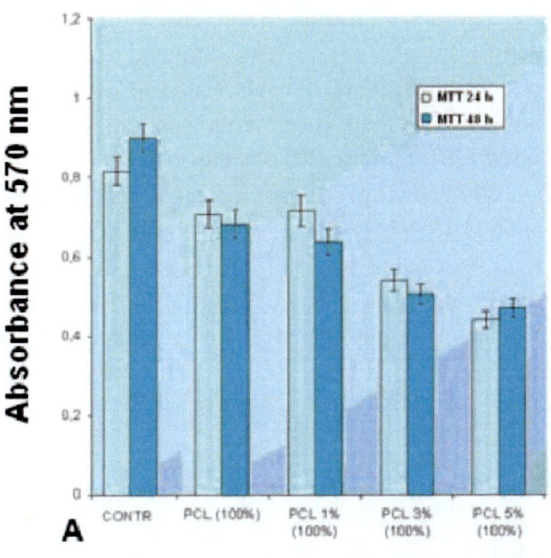

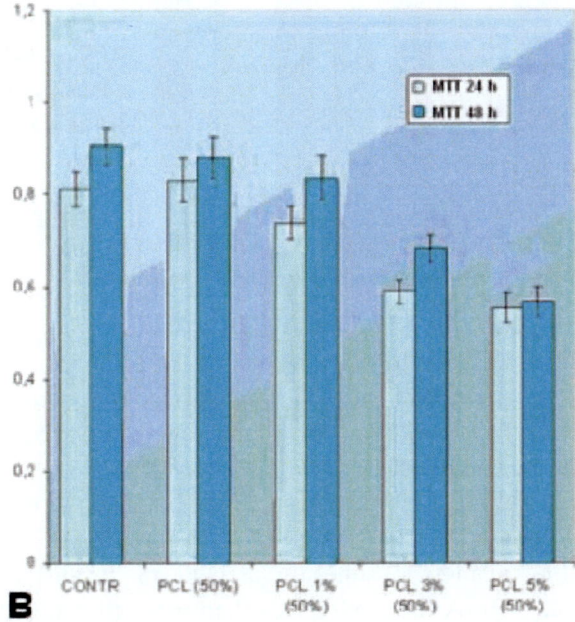

Figure 8. MTT test on 3T3 fibroblasts incubated for 24 and 48 h in presence of either 100% (A) or 50% (B) mechanical alloys extracts.

The composite samples (21 mm diameter-0.1 mm thickness) were cut in semilunar form with a surface of 3.6 cm^2, attached with bioinert silicon on the bottom of polystyrene 12-multiwell plates (surface of each well = 4 cm^2) and sterilized 24 h as indicated in the Experimental section.

The 0.4-cm^2 area left uncovered from the sample was intended to allow the observation of the cells growing in the immediate proximity of the materials. In fact, they were opaque to microscopic observation due to their semicrystalline nature. Each material was tested at least in triplicate.

MSCs were seeded on discs at a density of 15,000 cells/cm^2 and incubated at 37°C in a 5% CO_2 humidified atmosphere. Cell vitality at 24 hours were assessed by MTT test (Figure 9).

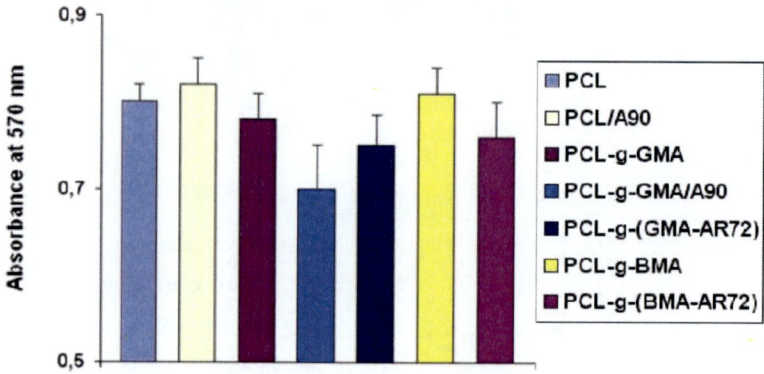

Figure 9. MTT test carried out 24 h after plating 60,000 MSCs ontoPCL (control) and its new derivatives and composites. The reported values result from the average of three analyses, each performed in triplicate.

The reported values were directly related to the affinity of cells towards the materials. It was apparent that the adhesion varied in a narrow range from a minimum of 0.70 for PCL-g-GMA/A90 to a maximum of 0.82 for PCL/A90 with a value of 0.80 for the control PCL.

After 7-days of culture, MTT test was carried out again in order to assess cell growth on the various materials (Figure 10). The proliferation pattern reflected and overlapped that relative to adhesion of cells to the different discs, being PCL/A90 and PCL-g-BMA the composites that, more than others, had favoured the adhesion and then the cell growth.

Realization and Performance Analysis of PCL/ Silica Nanocomposites... 27

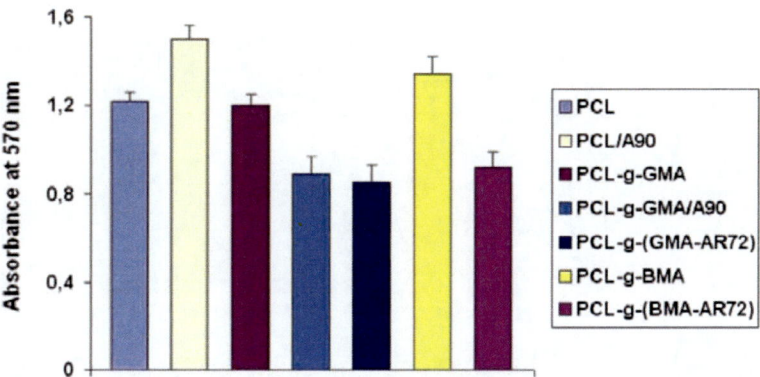

Figure 10. MTT test carried out 7 days after plating 60,000 MSCs onto PCL (control) and its new derivatives and composites. The reported values result from the average of three experiments, each performed in triplicate.

Figure 11 shows the macroscopic appearance of discs of PCL-g-BMA and PCL-g-GMA and of their corresponding biocomposites with functionalised nanosilica AR72. A substantial and regular cell colonization was evident on both PCL-g-BMA and PCL-g-GMA, whereas on their AR72-derivatives composites cells were not only quantitatively lesser but also unevenly distributed.

In addition, crystal violet staining performed in parallel confirmed the minor presence of the cells with respect to composites containing AR72 nanosilica (Figure 12).

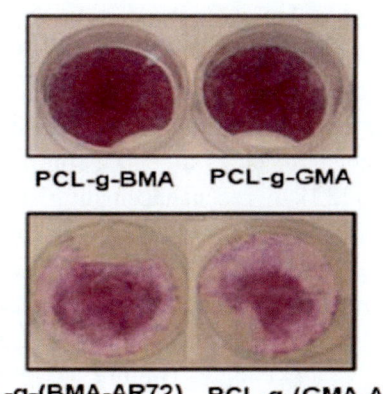

Figure 11. The macroscopic appearance of some PCL composites after MTT test carried out 7 days after cell seeding.

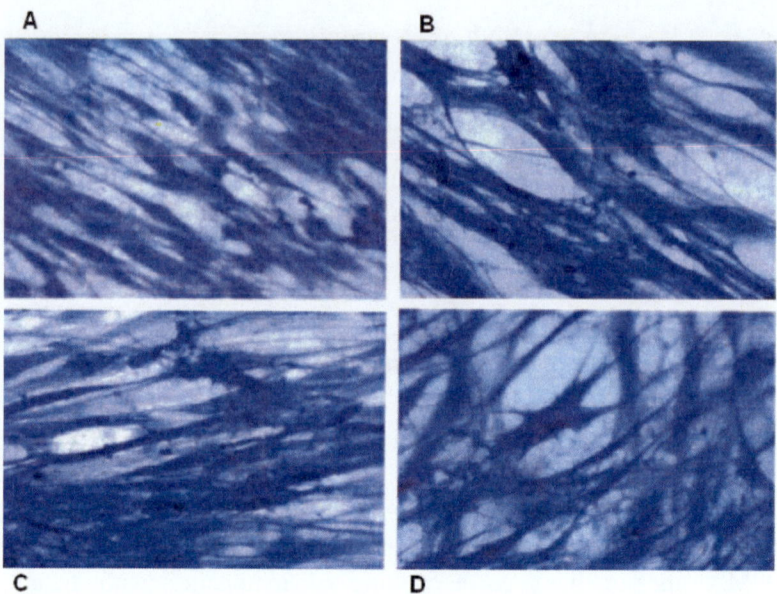

Figure 12. The microscopic appearance of MSCs cultured for 7 days on PCL-g-BMA (A), PCL-g-(BMA-AR72) (B), PCL-g-GMA (C), PCL-g-(GMA-AR72) (D), after crystal violet staining (Magnification 200x).

The differentiation of MSCs toward the osteoblastic phenotype is a complex process which follows a precise temporal sequence involving several phases [131]. Alkaline phosphatase (AP), commonly considered an early marker of osteogenic differentiation, is involved in the hydroxyapatite crystal deposition and hence in mineralization of extracellular collagenic matrix [132]. Osteocalcin is a specific late marker of osteogenic differentiation, representing the major non-collagenic protein of the bone matrix, and is expressed exclusively by cells of osteoblastic lineage. Osteocalcin plays a central role in bone mineralization and calcium ion homeostasis [133]. A recent fascinating study has demonstrated that this molecule can be actually considered a hormone by which skeleton exerts a feedback endocrine regulation of energy metabolism [134].

Therefore, to analyze the influence of the various materials on MSCs' differentiative pattern, the expression of the of the early and late osteoblastic markers, namely AP (Figure 13) and OC (Figure 14), at 7 and 14 days of culture, respectively, was assessed.

It was evident that PCL-g-BMA expressed the maximum value of alkaline phosphatase activity compared to PCL control, whereas its derivative composite

PCL-g-(BMA-AR72) exhibited values markedly lower. This decrease was even more pronounced in the case of PCL-g-GMA and PCL-g-(GMA-AR72).

On the contrary, the osteocalcin synthesis by MSCs cultured on both BMA- and GMA-derivatives composites exhibited values grater than the control PCL. In particular, it is to underline that high OC levels were expressed by cells grown on the two AR72-composites, in spite of the clearly minor presence of MSCs on these materials (Figures 9-11).

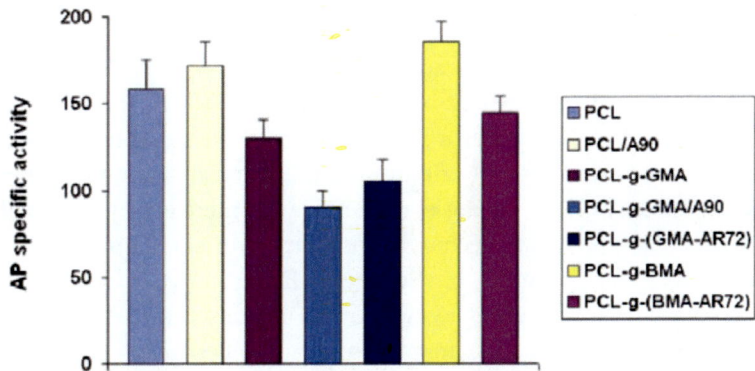

Figure 13. Alkaline phosphatase specific activity of stromal cells cultured for 7 days on PCL (control) and its new derivatives and composites. The reported values result from the average of three experiments, each performed in triplicate.

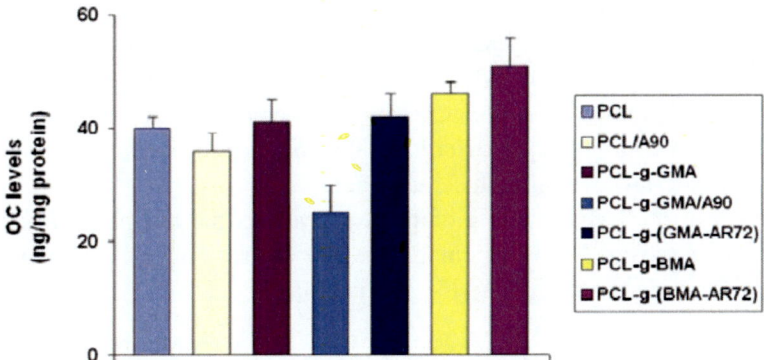

Figure 14. Osteocalcin synthesis 2 weeks after MSCs' plating on PCL (control) and its new derivatives and composites. The last three days the cells were incubated in FCS-free Opti-MEM in presence of 0.1% bovine serum albumin and 100 nM 1,25-dihydroxycholecalciferol. The reported values result from the average of three experiments, each performed in triplicate.

Conclusion

In this chapter we have reported the preparation and characterization of new composites based on polycaprolactone reinforced with nanostructured silica, projected for biomedical applications in orthopaedic, maxillo-facial and dental surgery fields.

The chemical modification of the PCL, necessary to realize a stable interface with the nanosilica, has been carried out directly in the processing equipment and has allowed to increase the mechanical characteristics of the polyester without worsening its biocompatibility characteristics.

The work has been carried out in two steps. In the first one, the characterization of mechanical properties performed on the new nanocomposites has demonstrated an increase of rigidity of the material without compromising the tenacity. In particular, Young's modulus was increased to a level by far superior to the neat PCL. The mechanical properties reflect the morphology of the materials, analyzed by means of Scanning Electron Microscopy, where an interfacial adhesion was clearly evidenced as a consequence of the chemical modification. In conclusion, the improvement of mechanical properties of the nanocomposites compared with the pure PCL can allow their potential use as scaffolds or membrane barriers.

In the second phase of our study we investigated in vitro the biocompatibility of these novel biocomposites as well as their capacity to induce the osteogenic differentiation of human bone marrow stromal cells. In particular we analyzed the adhesion and the growth of these cells, being the contact with the material crucial for all the following events, including the expression of biochemical specific markers, namely alkaline phosphatase and osteocalcin. None of new PCL-silica nanocomposites exhibited cytotoxicity, on the contrary the cells adhered and grew onto all the materials even if at different extent.

Overall, at the basis of the biological as well as the mechanical results, the novel nanocomposites, in particular the one based on PCL-g-BMA, appear promising for bone tissue engineering applications.

EXPERIMENTAL

Materials

Poly-ε-caprolactone (PCL) CAPA® 650, molecular weight 50.000 m.a.u., was a gentle gift from Solvay (Italy).

Nanostructured silica Aerosil® 90, as well as functionalised nanostructured silica Aerosil® R7200, were a kind gift from Degussa.

Dibenzoylperoxide (DBPO) is a Sigma Aldrich product.

Glycidylmethacrylate (GMA) and butylmethacrylate (BMA) are Fluka reagent grade products.

All cell culture biologics were purchased from (Life Technologies, MD, USA), and all chemicals were from Sigma Chemical Co (St. Louis, MO, USA) when not otherwise specified.

Murine fibroblasts NIH 3T3 were from ATCC (LGC Milano).

PREPARATION OF SILICA NANOPARTICLES

Silica nanoparticles were prepared by using the Stöber methodology. The method consists in a hydrolysis reaction followed by a polycondensation catalyzed by an alkaline water solution of tetraethoxysilane (TEOS). The process is hereafter summarized:

a) hydrolysis:

$$Si(OEt)_4 + 4 H_2O \xrightarrow{^-OH} Si(OH)_4 + 4 EtOH$$

b) polycondensation:

$$Si(OH)_4 \longrightarrow SiO_2 + 2 H_2O$$

or

$$Si(OH)_4 + Si(OEt)_4 \longrightarrow SiO_2 + 4 EtOH$$

PREPARATION OF NANOCOMPOSITES

A. Mechanical Alloys

Before the realization of the functionalized nanocomposites, mechanical alloys based on matrix PCL with a percentage of silica of 1, 3 and 5% have been prepared. The silica employed was Aerosil® 90 (A90). At first three different mixtures have been prepared in the following proportions:

- Mechanical alloy PCL/A90 1% = 49.5 g of PCL + 0.5 g of A90
- Mechanical alloy PCL/A90 3% = 48.5 g of PCL + 1.5 g of A90
- Mechanical alloy PCL/A90 5% = 47.5 g of PCL + 2,5 g of A90

The preparation of the material has been made in a static mixer type Brabender (Rheocord) to a temperature of 100°C and for a time of 10 minutes, 8 rpm for the first 5 minutes and then 32 rpm for the remaining time. 1,5 g of the material thus obtained have been compression moulded to a temperature of 100°C for 3 minutes and to a pressure of 5 Kg/cm^2, in order to obtain a film having the dimensions of approximately 10x10cm and a thickness between 80 and 100 µm.

B. Functionalised Nanocomposites

For allowing a direct comparison, the nanocomposites have been realized having the same percentages of nanosilica of mechanical alloys that is, 1, 3 and 5%. It has been employed the functionalised silica Aerosil® R7200 (AR72) with a vinyl end group. Moreover the PCL has been *in situ* functionalised with glycidylmethacrylate (GMA) using dibenzoylperoxide (DBPO) as radical source. The three different mixtures have been prepared in the following proportions:

- nanocomposite PCL-g-(GMA-AR72 1%) = 49.5g of PCL + 0.5g of AR72 + 0.495g DBPO + 4.95g of GMA
- nanocomposite PCL-g-(GMA-AR72 3%) = 48.5g of PCL + 1.5g of AR72 + 0.485g DBPO + 4.85g of GMA
- nanocomposite PCL-g-(GMA-AR72 5%) = 47.5g of PCL + 2.5g of AR72 + 0.475g DBPO + 4.75g of GMA

The preparation has been made in a static mixer type Brabender (Rheocord) initially to a temperature of 100°C for 10 minutes in order to obtain the formation of the GMA functionalised PCL and then for further 10 min to graft the functionalised silica on the PCL previously obtained (reactive mixing) progressively increasing the number of turns from 8 to 32 rpm. Also for these materials films have been prepared as previously described.

As reference and control materials also the following samples have been prepared:

- PCL functionalised with 1% GMA (PCL-g-GMA)
- PCL functionalised with GMA + silica A90 1% (PCL-g-GMA/A90 1%)

DIFFERENTIAL THERMAL ANALYSIS (DSC)

Differential thermal analysis on polymer matrix (PCL) has been carried out using the following thermal cycle: heating of the sample from 30 to 180°C at a scanning speed of 10°C/min then cooling to - 100°C to the scanning speed of 10°C/min and successive heating till 180°C to the same scanning speed. The nanocomposites have been subjected to the same thermal cycle. The calorimeter used was Mettler DSC 30.

Mechanical Tests

Tensile mechanical tests have been performed on samples in the form of dog's bone just like the norm prescribes, and tested in traction in order to obtain relevant mechanical parameters. The tests have been carried out on a Instron dynamometer model 4505 at room temperature with a traction speed of 10mm/sec. The analyses have been performed on previously described mechanical alloys and nanocomposites.

SCANNING AND TRANSMISSION ELECTRON MICROSCOPY (SEM AND TEM)

The morphology of the materials has been evaluated examining the fracture surfaces by SEM. The samples were fractured in liquid nitrogen, mounted on a support and metallized with a Au/Pd alloy. The microscope used was a Philips XL 20.

TEM allowed the observation of the as obtained silica nanoparticles. The nanoparticles were collected from a water suspension directly onto TEM supports and observed. The microscope used was a Philips EM 430.

Elution Test

The samples, in form of thin layers, were first sterilized in a steam autoclave and then placed in a suitable ratio weight/volume of Dulbecco's modified Eagle's medium (0.1 g/ml medium) containing penicillin (100 units/ml), streptomycin (100 µg/ml) and fungizone (1.2 µg/ml), and left under stirring at room temperature either for 24 or for 48 hours. The corresponding extracts were added, as such (100%) or diluted 1:1 (50%), to confluent 3T3 cells, that had been plated two days before in multiwell-12. The cultures were incubated at 37°C in a 5% CO_2 humidified atmosphere and cell vitality at 24 and 48 hours was assessed by MTT test.

PREPARATION AND CHARACTERIZATION OF BONE MARROW MSCs

The preparation of MSCs was performed employing heparinized human bone marrow from healthy volunteers, after informed consent, following the method of Friedenstein et al. with some modifications [12,135]. Taking into account that a number of factors, as the donor-to-donor variability, age, gender, etc, might affect the biological response, four different MSCs populations were obtained in order to enhance data reliability.

Briefly, the bone marrow sample was diluted 1:5 with Opti-MEM (Life Technologies, MD, USA), containing 10% fetal calf serum (FCS), penicillin 100 units/ml, streptomycin 100 µg/ml and sodium ascorbate 50 µg/ml (growth medium), placed in 100 mm polystyrene dishes and incubated at 37°C in a 5% CO_2 humidified atmosphere.

After 48 h, the medium was collected and centrifuged at 800 rpm. Half of the supernatant (conditioned medium, CM) was aspirated, added with an equal volume of fresh medium and placed in the first plate. The medium remaining in the tube was used to resuspend the cellular pellet and, after the addition of an equivalent volume of fresh culture medium, the entire cellular suspension was plated in a second dish. The day after, also the medium of the second plate was centrifuged: the pellet, containing all non-adherent cellular elements, was discarded while the corresponding CM was added again to the dish.

In 2-4 days, several foci of adherent spindle-like cells started to appear and to develop until to colonize the whole dish surface in the following two weeks. During this period fresh medium was added every 3 days, each time leaving one half of the old medium. After the reaching of the confluence, cells were trypsinized and amplified always diluting the conditioned medium.

MSCs were the analyzed by flow cytometry using a wide panel of monoclonal antibodies. The cells expressed specific surface markers, such as CD13, CD29, CD44, CD105, CD166, and were negative for hematopoietic cell markers CD14, CD34 and CD45.

Cultures between the 3rd and 5th passage were used in our experiments. The cells harvested from each donor were kept separately and not pooled with other preparations.

In presence of osteogenic inducers, the stromal cells go through a complex series of events, at the end of which the multipotent cells become terminally differentiated. Alkaline phosphatase and osteocalcin are phenotypic markers for early-stage differentiated and terminally differentiated osteoblasts, respectively.

DIRECT CONTACT TEST

The samples, in form of discs (21 mm diameter and 0.1 mm thickness), were attached with biological silicone (NuSil Silicone Technology, CA, USA) to the bottom of 12-well plates and sterilized 24 h with PBS containing penicillin (1000 units/ml), streptomycin (1000 µg/ml) and fungizone (12.5 µg/ml) at 37°C in a 5% CO_2 humidified atmosphere. The materials were then placed in Opti-MEM containing antibiotics and fungizone (at concentrations ten-fold lower than those indicated above), 10% FCS and 50 µg/ml sodium ascorbate (complete medium) and kept in the incubator overnight before plating the cells.

MSCs were seeded on discs at a density of 15,000 cells/cm^2 in complete culture medium and incubated for up to 2 weeks at 37°C in a 5% CO_2 humidified atmosphere. Cell adhesion and vitality, as well as alkaline phosphatase activity and osteocalcin levels were evaluated.

MTT Test

The MTT assay is a very simple and useful tool for evaluating cell vitality and proliferation. The key component is 3-(4,5-dimethylthiazol-2-yl)-2,5-diphenyltetrazolium bromide (MTT). Mitochondrial dehydrogenases of living cells reduced the tetrazolium ring, yielding a blue formazan product, which was measured spectrophotometrically. The amount of formazan produced is proportional to the number of viable cells present. MTT (5 mg/ml in DMEM without phenol red) was added to the wells in an amount equivalent to 10% of the culture medium. After an incubation of 4 h at 37°C, the liquid was aspirated and the insoluble formazan produced was dissolved in isopropanol. The optical densities were measured at 570 nm, subtracting background absorbance determined at 690 nm.

ALKALINE PHOSPHATASE ASSAY

After the removal of the medium, the wells were rinsed with 20 mM TRIS HCl-0.5 M NaCl, pH 7.4 (TBS) and the cells were solubilized with lysis buffer, that is TBS containing DTT (0.5 mM), PMSF (0.5 mM) and Triton X-100 (0.25%). After 30 min in ice, the cell lysates were centrifuged at 12,000g for 5 min, and the supernatants assayed for alkaline phosphatase activity. The protein concentration was determined using the protein assay kit (Bio-Rad Laboratories, CA, USA), according to the method of Bradford.

AP activity was determined by measuring the release of p-nitrophenol from disodium p-nitrophenyl phosphate (PNPP). The reaction mixture contained 0.1 M diethanolamine buffer, pH 10.5, 0.5mM $MgCl_2$ and 12 mM PNPP in a final volume of 0.5 ml. The reaction was initiated by the addition of the cell extract and the mixture was incubated at 37°C for 30 min. The reaction was stopped by adding 0.5 ml of 0.5 M NaOH and the absorbance was determined spectrophotometrically at 405 nm. The AP activity was normalized to the protein content and expressed as units/mg protein, where one unit was defined as the amount of enzyme that hydrolyzes 1 nmol of PNPP/min under the specified conditions.

OSTEOCALCIN SYNTHESIS

To evaluate osteocalcin synthesis, confluent cultures grown on the different surfaces for 2 weeks were incubated in FCS-free Opti-MEM in presence of 0.1% bovine serum albumin and 100 nM 1,25- dihydroxycholecalciferol for 48 h. The levels of polypeptide secreted in the medium were measured by means of an immunoenzymatic assay (Biosource International, Camarillo, CA, USA) that utilizes monoclonal highly specific antibodies and a peroxidase as conjugated enzyme. The amount of osteocalcin was calculated in ng/ml and then normalized to the protein content.

STATISTICAL ANALYSIS

All the experiments were performed in triplicate on at least two different cell preparations. Data are expressed as the mean ± standard deviation (SD) of values. The means of each experimental group were compared by unpaired Student's t-test, with the value of significance set at $P < 0.05$.

Chapter 3

NOVEL INJECTABLE ALGINATE/ N-SUCCINYLCHITOSAN/CALCIUM SULPHATE COMPOSITES AS BONE-DEFECTS FILLERS

Giovanna Gomez d'Ayala, Paola Laurienzo, Mario Malinconico, Adriana Oliva

A preformed scaffold might not conform to the irregular shape and size of a bone defect when implanted in the body. At the double aim to overcome this limitation and to minimize the invasivity of the surgical approach, injectable scaffolds have been designed [136].

These systems can be stored for a long time in form of soft putty-like constructs without losing their peculiarity, that is just the injectability. Once injected in the defect, the material hardens making a porous and biodegradable structure that the cells at the site of bone defect can colonize finding in situ the appropriate environment in terms of cytokines and growth factors. A more promising alternative to this approach could consist in encapsulating stem cells and bioactive molecules in the injectable paste: after the injection and the hardening of the material, the cells and the growth factors are directly delivered to the site of bone repair.

At the aim to project a new injectable scaffold for bone tissue engineering application, Gomez d'Ayala *et al.* [127, 137] developed a novel composite based on blends of alginate and a modified chitosan, N-succinylchitosan, containing calcium sulphate as mineral osteoinductive phase. It has been demonstrated that the action mechanism of calcium sulphate (CHS) occurs through the dissolution of the low soluble salt and the local precipitation of calcium phosphate (CP), due to the increase of calcium ion concentration and its contact with body fluids. The CP deposits conduce bone cells into the defect and accelerate tissue regeneration [122,124]. Therefore, it is necessary that the salt dissolution rate is compatible with bone growth inside the defect, in order to allow bone regeneration before the substitute completely disappears. Encapsulation of calcium sulphate into a slowly biodegradable polymer matrix represents a solution to the problem, as allows to slow down the salt dissolution, increasing the time of its permanence inside the bone defect.

Alginate (Alg) and chitosan (Ch) were chosen as component of the polymeric matrix because of their biocompatibility and adequate biodegradability. Unlike chitosan scaffolds, which can only be fabricated from acidic solutions, the chitosan-alginate scaffolds can be prepared from solutions at physiological or basic pH, which provide favourable environment for incorporating growth factors or proteins (as cytokines) with less risk of denaturation. Bone forming osteoblastic cells attached readily to chitosan-alginate scaffolds, proliferated well, and deposited calcified matrix [58] Moreover, in order to obtain a homogeneous paste in presence of water, chitosan was previously modified with succinic anhydride to get a water-soluble polymer, according to a previously reported procedure [85].

The succinylation reaction (illustrated in the scheme 1) consists of a condensation reaction between the polysaccharide amine group and the electrophilic carbonyl group of anhydride. The reaction involves the formation of an amidic bond with opening of the anhydride ring, which causes the introduction of acid carboxylic functions onto chitosan chains. It was necessary to dissolve the pristine chitosan in an acidic solution, because of its insolubility in water.

However, in this condition amine groups of polymer are protonated and consequently their nucleophilicity is adversely affected.therefore, in order to preserve their nucleophilicity, a higher value of pH was necessary. As the final modified chitosan (sCh) was found to be soluble at pH 7, the pH of reaction solution was continuously adjusted to this value by a slow and simultaneous dropwise addition of NaOH solution, in order to avoid the chitosan precipitation in the course of the reaction.

Scheme 1. Succinylation reaction of chitosan.

Solubility tests were carried out in order to compare the behaviour of the two polymers at different pH values in aqueous solutions. In Figure 15 the solubility curves of both pristine and modified polymers are shown as a function of the pH. In the investigated pH range the two polymers showed an opposite behaviour in terms of solubility, as expected. In fact, sCh is completely soluble in the range of pH between 6 and 12.

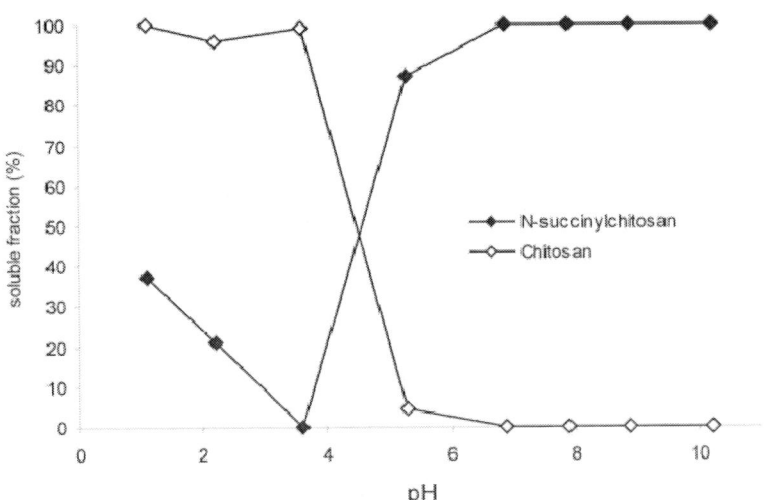

* Reprinted from *J. Biomed. Mat. Res, Part A, 81*, Development of a new calcium sulphate-based composite using alginate and chemically modified chitosan for bone regeneration, p. 817, Copyright 2007, with permission from Wiley.

Figure 15*. Solubility (% by weight) vs pH of chitosan and N-succinylchitosan. (Note: caption should be at bottom of page 41)

To prepare the composites, finely grounded hemihydrate calcium sulphate, Alg and sCh powders were mixed in different compositions. The composite was prepared by adding dropwise distilled water to the mixture until the resulting paste became fully wet (1.8 ml of water each 1.5 g of material). The addition of water to the powder mixture promotes the transformation of calcium sulphate from the hemihydrate form to the dihydrate one. During this process calcium ions are available for the crosslinking of alginate. The setting of the materials is due to the transformation of the hemihydrate calcium sulphate into the dihydrate form and partially to the cross-linking of alginate with calcium ions. As a matter of fact, a mouldable and easy-to-spread paste, which get a hard cement in few hours, was obtained. This allows the material to be easily handled and moulded into the desired shape and to turn into a hard cement in a short setting time (2 hours).

Mechanical analyses in compression mode were performed on composites constituted by a fixed amount of CHS and variable ratios of the other two components and for sake of comparison on a composite in which N-succinylchitosan was substituted by plain chitosan. The results, shown in **Table 5**, demonstrated that the blend of alginate and N-succinylchitosan causes a substantial reinforcement of composite.

Table 5. Yield strength and Young modulus (± STD) of composites with calcium sulphate and variable amounts of the polymeric components (Alg: Alginate; Ch: Chitosan; sCh: N-succinylchitosan)

Sample	Yield strength (MPa)	Young's Modulus (MPa)
CHS/Alg: 50/50	0,03 ± 0,01	20,2 ± 3,5
CHS/sCh: 50/50	0,80 ± 0,21	14,7 ± 4,3
CHS/Alg/sCh: 50/10/40	4,58 ± 1,63	427,4 ± 79,8
CHS/Alg/sCh: 50/20/30	13,62 ± 0,41	873,9 ± 145,8
CHS/Alg/sCh: 50/25/25	8,20 ± 0,15	370,8 ± 73,7
CHS/Alg/sCh: 50/30/20	9,02 ± 2,62	437,9 ± 83,5
CHS/Alg/sCh: 50/40/10	3,22 ± 0,59	444,2 ± 74,7
CHS/Alg/Ch: 50/30/20	0,04 ± 0,01	9,9 ± 0,6

In fact, by comparing mechanical properties of CHS/Alg/sCh composite with those of plain chitosan-based composite, it has been observed that in presence of the modified chitosan the mechanical performance is largely improved. It seems that the carboxylic groups grafted onto the chitosan modified chain, in addition to those of alginate, enhance the chelating power of the polysaccharide mixture because of an additional synergistic effect with respect to the classic "egg-box" effect of alginate (Figure 16) [138]:

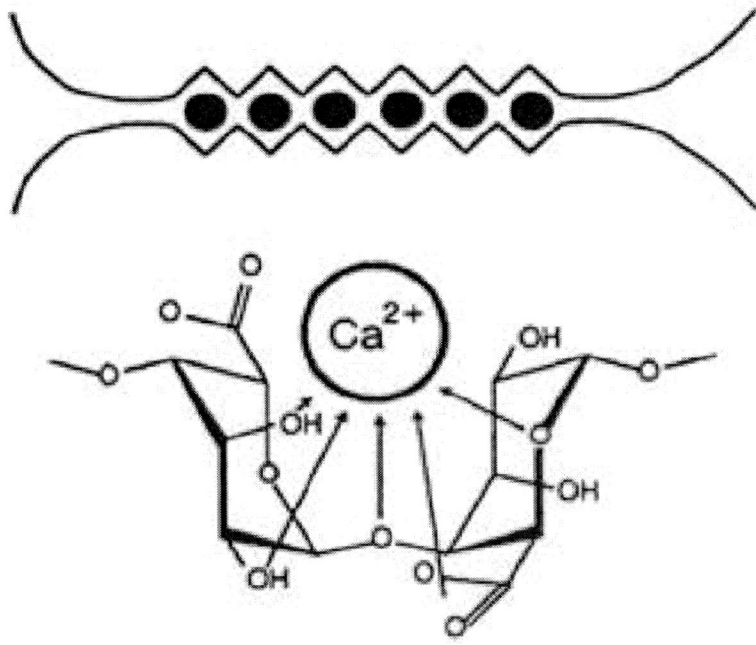

Figure 16. Egg-box model for the cross-linking of alginate with calcium ions.

This was demonstrated also by a rheological study of a blend of plain alginate and N-succinyl-chitosan polymers in presence of a slow release calcium ions source [137]. This study showed that, in favourable conditions of concentration and composition, most of the chitosan molecules can effectively interact with the alginate network and might co-crosslink with alginate through calcium ions. A significant acceleration of the gelation kinetic observed for a given alginate/N-succinylchitosan composition, with respect to the case of the plain alginate gel, confirmed the hypothesis of a synergistic effect of the N-succinylchitosan in chelating calcium ions during the alginate gelation process.

Besides, morphological analyses showed that calcium sulphate crystals are embedded into the cross-linked polymer matrix with scarce evidence of discontinuity between the polymeric components and the inorganic filler (Figure 17). This could depend on the presence on both polymer chains of negatively charged carboxylic groups, which allow a stronger interaction with calcium ions.

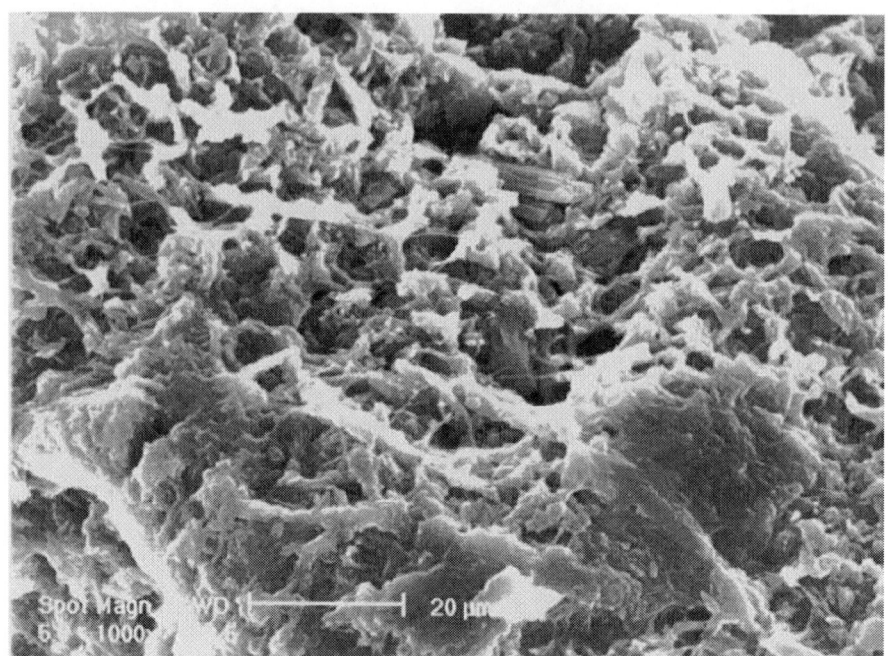

* Reprinted from *J. Biomed. Mat. Res, Part A, 81*, Development of a new calcium sulphate-based composite using alginate and chemically modified chitosan for bone regeneration, p. 817, Copyright 2007, with permission from Wiley.

Figure 17*. Scanning electron micrographs of CHS/Alg/sCh composite.

BIOLOGICAL EVALUATION

Biological assays were performed on a CHS/Alg/sCh 50/30/20 composite as such or with the addition of 10% demineralized bone matrix (DBM) (CHS/DBM/Alg/sCh 40/10/30/20).

To test *in vitro* the effect of this material on the biological response of MSCs, we made it to harden and then analyzed its influence on the growth and differentiation of bone marrow stromal cells. The samples, in form of little chips, derived from the mincing of the materials, were first autoclaved and then placed in a suitable ratio weight/volume of Opti-MEM (4 mg/ml medium) containing penicillin (100 units/ml), streptomycin (100 µg/ml) and fungizone (1.2 µg/ml), and left under agitation at room temperature for 24 hours.

This remarkable difference between the ratio weight/volume selected for the blends composites, compared to the above mentioned PCL-nanocomposites, is justified by the fast breaking up of the blends in aqueous environment forming a lot of tiny fragments that, in turn, are responsible for a large surface exchange between the materials and the medium.

The corresponding extracts were centrifuged at 15,000xg for 20 min and the supernatants added (100%) to semiconfluent cultures of bone marrow MSCs. As control extract we used medium complete added with calcium sulphate (1,8 mg/ml). After 7 day-culture at 37°C in a 5% CO_2 humidified atmosphere, MSCs vitality was assessed by MTT assay (Figure 18) and cell morphology was evaluated by crystal violet staining (Figure 19).

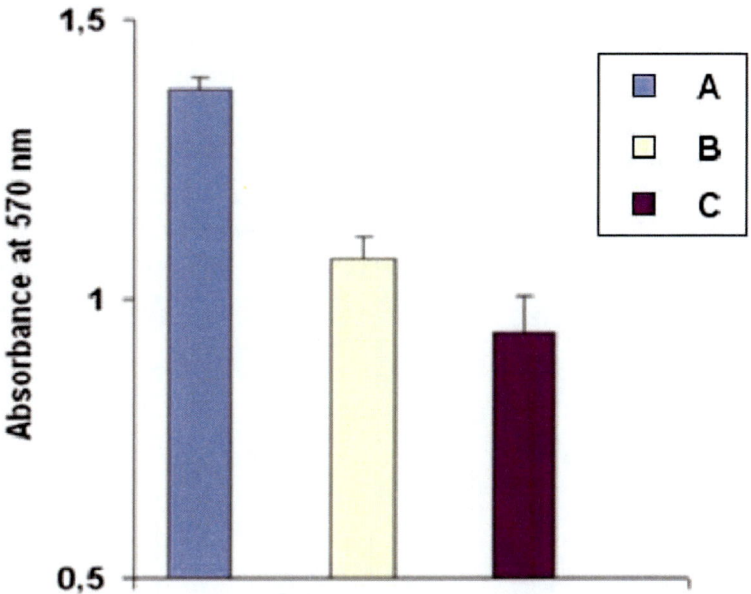

Figure 18. MTT test performed on MSCs incubated for 7 days in presence of complete medium added with: A = 1.8 mg/ml calcium sulphate; B = 4 mg/ml CHS/Alg/sCh (50/30/20); C = 4 mg/ml CHS/DBM/Alg/sCh (40/10/30/20). The reported values result from the average of three experiments, each performed in triplicate.

As shown in Fig. 18, the proliferation of cells in presence of each extract was clearly lesser than control, especially with respect to DBM-containing material. In the latter case, to the minor cell growth corresponded a more differentiated morphology, namely a polygonal shape of the MSCs.

In addition, the effects on osteogenic differentiation was evaluated analyzing the expression of alkaline phosphatase and osteocalcin, as well as the extracellular matrix mineralization.

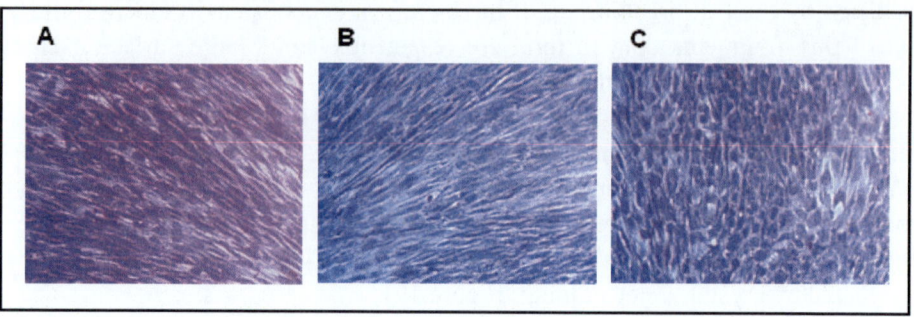

Figure 19. The microscopic appearance of MSCs cultured for 7 days in complete medium added with: A = 1.8 mg/ml calcium sulphate; B = 4 mg/ml CHS/Alg/sCh (50/30/20); C = 4 mg/ml CHS/DBM/Alg/sCh (40/10/30/20), after crystal violet staining (Magnification 100x).

Alkaline phosphatase was expressed at the highest value with CHS/DBM/Alg/sCh, at an intermediate value with CHS/Alg/sCh, while the lowest value matched with the highest cell growth extent of the control containing only calcium sulphate (Figure 20). Thus, the least cell growth corresponded a to more differentiated polygonal morphology, that in turn matched with the highest value of expression of AP.

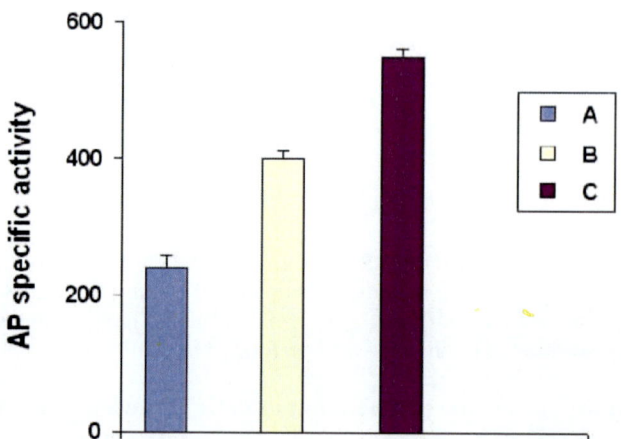

Figure 20. Alkaline phosphatase specific activity of stromal cells cultured for 7 days in complete medium added with: A = 1.8 mg/ml calcium sulphate; B = 4 mg/ml CHS/Alg/sCh (50/30/20); C = 4 mg/ml CHS/DBM/Alg/sCh (40/10/30/20). The reported values result from the average of three experiments, each performed in triplicate.

In addition, the effect on osteoblastic differentiation was evaluated analyzing the osteocalcin levels (Figure 21). It was evident that cells cultured in presence of the extract derived from CHS/DBM/Alg/sCh expressed OC values similar to the control, whereas the highest amount of osteocalcin was expressed by MSCs grown in the presence of CHS/DBM/Alg/sCh extract.

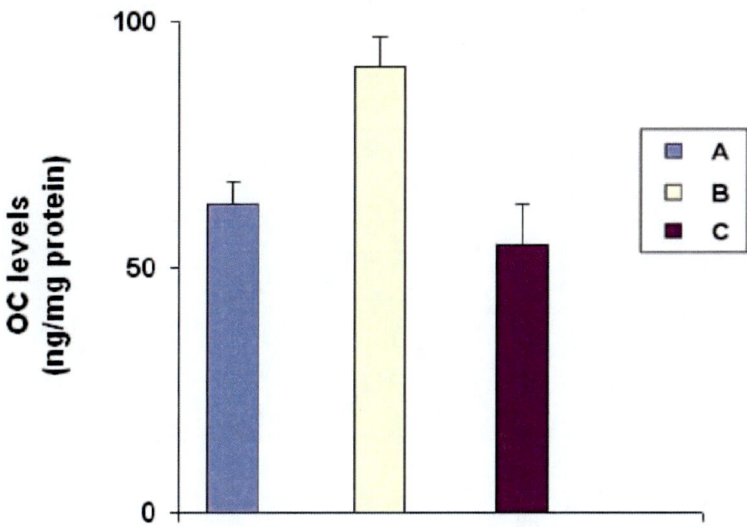

Figure 21. Osteocalcin synthesis after 2 weeks MSCs' culture in medium added with: A = 1.8 mg/ml calcium sulphate; B = 4 mg/ml CHS/Alg/sCh (50/30/20); C = 4 mg/ml CHS/DBM/Alg/sCh (40/10/30/20). The last three days the cells were incubated in FCS-free Opti-MEM in presence of 0.1% bovine serum albumin and 100 nM 1,25-dihydroxycolecalciferol. The reported values result from the average of three experiments, each performed in triplicate. (Note: caption should be at bottom of page 47)

After 3 week-culture in the presence of the extracts (changing the medium every 3 days), a staining with crystal violet was performed (Figure 22). It was apparent that, parallel to the higher proliferation, a dense network of collagen fibers covered up and hidden the control cells, while the cellular elements were more clearly distinguishable in the presence of each extract.

Finally, the extracellular matrix mineralization was tested by the quantification of the calcium levels. MSCs cultures were incubated for 2 weeks in the presence of the extracts and for the following 14 days in the presence an osteogenic medium composed of 100 nM dexamethasone and 10 mM β-glycerophosphate. Then, Alizarin Red assay showed a remarkably more intense and spread staining in control culture, whereas separate calcification nodules were apparent in extract-treated cells (Figure 23).

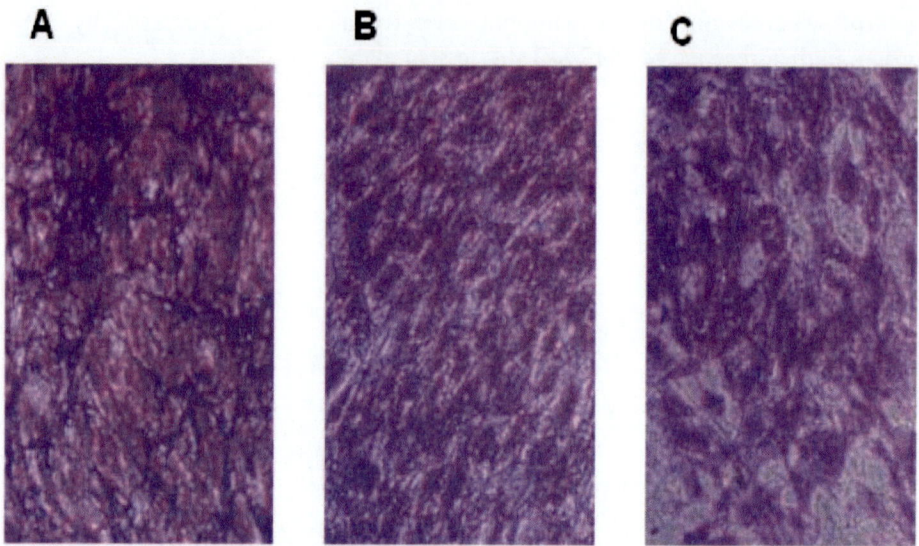

Figure 22. The microscopic appearance of MSCs cultured for 3 weeks in complete medium added with: A = 1.8 mg/ml calcium sulphate; B = 4 mg/ml CHS/Alg/sCh (50/30/20); C = 4 mg/ml CHS/DBM/Alg/sCh (40/10/30/20), after crystal violet staining (Magnification 100x).

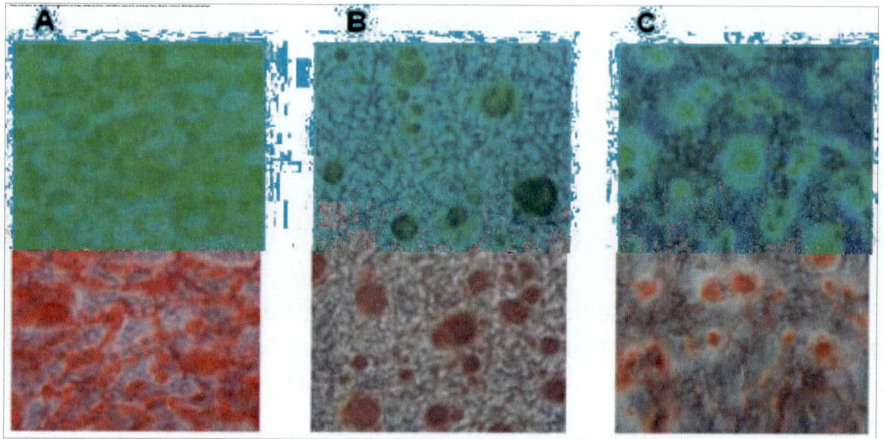

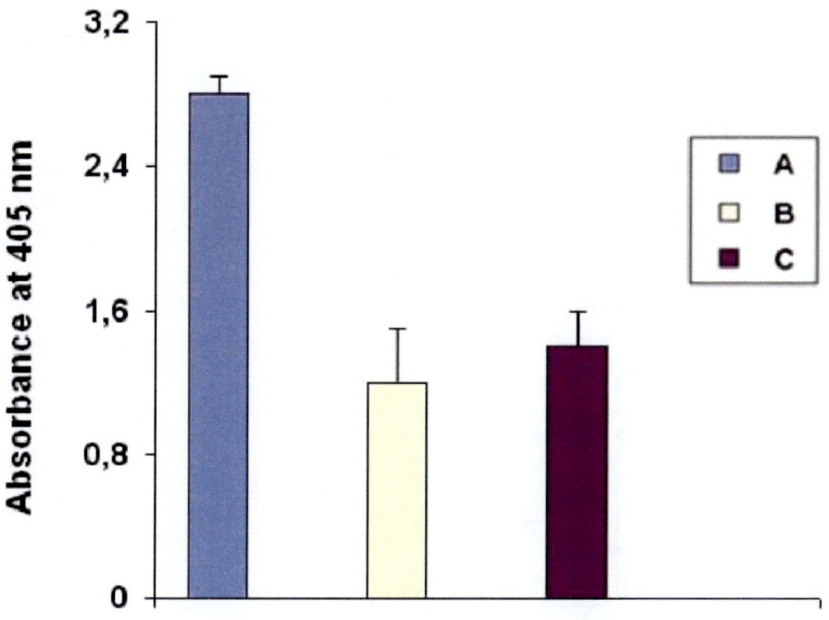

Figure 23. Alizarin Red staining. MSCs were cultured for 14 days in complete medium added with: A = 1.8 mg/ml calcium sulphate; B = 4 mg/ml CHS/Alg/sCh (50/30/20); C = 4 mg/ml CHS/DBM/Alg/sCh (40/10/30/20). For the following 2 weeks the cells were incubated in the presence of an osteogenic medium (100 nM dexamethasone - 10 mM β-glycerophosphate). First panel: microscopic appearance of cells (Magnification 100x). Second panel: quantification of matrix mineralization.

Conclusion

Calcium sulphate was encapsulated in a biodegradable polymeric matrix in order to prolong its structural integrity and slow-down its resorption. The analyses performed on the new material demonstrate that it should be suitable for biomedical applications and easy to use for the clinicians. In fact, the paste obtained by adding water to the powders mixture of the components shows a putty-like consistency and can be easily moulded to the desired shape.

Our results have demonstrated that the blend of alginate and N-succinylchitosan exhibited a substantial reinforcement of the corresponding obtained composite CHS/Alg/sCh, as a remarkable improvement of the mechanical performance compared with that of the plain alginate/chitosan- based composite (CHS/Alg/Ch) was found.

The addition of 10% demineralised bone matrix was also considered, in order to improve the osteoinductive potential of the composite.

As regards the biological features, assessed by elution test, it was evident that both formulations (Alg/sCh/CHS and Alg/sCh/DBM/CHS/) decreased cell growth, but in parallel greatly increased the osteogenic expression. In particular, the cells cultured in the presence of Alg/sCh/CHS, compared with control cells, expressed higher levels of the early marker AP, and levels even greater of the late marker OC. Furthermore, the extracellular matrix, even if apparently less rich of collagen fibers, was able to mineralize and to produce calcific nodules.

These encouraging results support the potential applications of the novel N-succinylchitosan/alginate-based injectable scaffolds as an improved alternative to other natural polymer-based scaffolds for tissue engineering applications.

EXPERIMENTAL

Materials

Medium molecular weight Chitosan (Ch), medium molecular weight Sodium Alginate (Alg) and Succinic Anhydride (SA) were all purchased from Fluka-Aldrich and used as received.

Hemihydrate calcium sulphate (CHS) was kindly provided by ClassImplant s.r.l., Rome, Italy.

Demineralized bone matrix (DBM) was purchased from Integra Orthobiologics, Irvine (CA), USA.

Pyridine, purchased from Fluka, was distilled under reduced pressure prior to use.

All the solvents were of analytical grade.

All cell culture biologics were purchased from (Life Technologies, MD, USA), and all chemicals were from Sigma Chemical Co (St. Louis, MO, USA) when not otherwise specified.

PREPARATION OF N-SUCCINYLCHITOSAN

To a 2% chitosan solution (w/v) in aqueous HCl (0,37%) a solution of succinic anhydride (SA) in pyridine (12,5% w/v) was dropwise added under vigorous stirring at room temperature (RT). SA was used in a 2:1 molar ratio with respect to chitosan. The pH of the reaction mixture was adjusted to 7,0 by simultaneously adding a NaOH solution (1,0M) dropwise. NaOH addition was continued until the pH was stabilized [52]. After 40 minutes of reaction, the modified polymer obtained was precipitated in a large excess of methanol, washed with acetone and desiccated. The as obtained product was finely grounded. In order to remove ungrafted SA, the resulting powder was dissolved and dialysed in a pH=10 NaOH solution for 48h using a dialysis membrane bag with a molecular weight cut-off of 10 kDa.

Mechanical Tests

Mechanical tests were performed on cylindrical samples (diameter 13 mm, height 15 cm) obtained by compression moulding the wet powder mixture at room temperature and by leaving it at room temperature for setting. Samples were then analysed in compressive mode at room temperature on an Instron dynamometer model 4505 at a cross-head speed of 1 mm/min.

Osteogenic Markers (AP, OC) Evaluation

The same protocol described in the case of PCL-silica nanocomposites has been adopted for these novel alginate/N-succinylchitosan/calcium sulphate composites.

Extracellular Matrix Mineralization

In order to induce extracellular matrix mineralization, control cells were cultured for 3 weeks in presence of osteogenic medium (culture medium supplemented with 10 mM β-glycerophosphate, 100 nM dexamethasone). At the end of this period, the calcium levels were measured colorimetrically using Alizarin Red Staining (ARS). Briefly, cell layers were washed with PBS, fixed in 10% formaldehyde for 15 min and then washed with dH_2O prior to adding 1 ml of 40 mM ARS (pH 4.1) per well. The plate was incubated for 20 min and then washed four times with dH2O. For quantification of staining, 800 μl 10% acetic acid was added to each well, and the plate was incubated at room temperature for 30 min with shaking. The cell layer was then scraped from the plate, collected together with the acetic acid and vortexed for 30 sec. The slurry was centrifuged at 20,000xg for 15 min and 500 µl of the supernatant was transferred into a new 1.5-ml microfuge tube. Then 200 µl of 10% ammonium hydroxide was added to neutralize the acid. Aliquots of the obtained solution were read in triplicate at 405 nm in 96-well.

REFERENCES

[1] Langer, R. & Vacanti, J.P. (1993). Tissue engineering. *Science,* 260, 920-6.
[2] MacArthur, B. & Oreffo, R.O.C. (2005). Bridging the gap. *Nature*, 433, 19.
[3] Friedenstein, A.J.; Chailakhyan, R.K. & Gerasimov, U.V. (1987). Bone marrow osteogenic stem cells: in vitro cultivation and transplantation in diffusion chambers. *Cell Tissue Kinet*, 20, 263-72.
[4] Prockop, D.J. (1997) Marrow stromal cells as stem cells for nonhematopoietic tissues. *Science*, 27, 671-74.
[5] Pittenger, M.F.; Mackay, A.M.; Beck, S.C.; Jaiswal, R.K.; Douglas, R.; Mosca, J.D.; Moorman, M.A.; Simonetti, D.W.; Craig, S. & Marshak, D.R. (1999). Multilineage potential of adult human mesenchymal stem cells. *Science*, 284, 143-147.
[6] Toma, C.; Pittenger, M.F.; Cahill, K.S.; Byrne, B.J. & Kessler, P.D. (2002). Human mesenchymal stem cells differentiate to a cardiomyocyte phenotype in the adult murine heart. *Circulation*, 105, 93-98.
[7] Kopen, G.C.; Prockop, D.J. & Phinney, D.G. (1999). Marrow stromal cells migrate throughout forebrain and cerebellum, and they differentiate into astrocytes after injection into neonatal mouse brains. *Proc. Natl. Acad. Sci. USA,* 96, 10711-16.
[8] Woodbury, D.; Schwarz, E.J.; Black, I.B. & Prockop, D.J. (2000). Adult rat and human bone marrow stromal cells differentiate into neurons. *Neurosci Res,* 61, 364-70.
[9] Seshi, B.; Kumar, S. & Sellers, D. (2000). Human bone marrow stromal cell: coexpression of markers specific for multiple mesenchymal cell lineages. *Blood Cells Mol. Dis.* 26, 234-46.
[10] Herzog, E.L.; Chai, L. & Krause, D.S. (2003). Plasticity of marrow-derived stem cells. *Blood.* 102, 3483-93.

[11] Di Nicola, M.; Carlo-Stella, C.; Magni, M.; Milanesi, M.; Longoni, P.D.; Matteucci, P.; Grisanti, S. & Gianni, A.M. (2002). Human bone marrow stromal cells suppress T-lymphocyte proliferation induced by cellular or nonspecific mitogenic stimuli. *Blood*, 99, 3838-3843.

[12] Oliva, A.; Passaro, I.; Di Pasquale, R.; Di Feo, A.; Criscuolo, M.; Zappia, V.; Della Ragione, F.; D'Amato, S.; Annunziata, M. & Guida, L. (2005). Ex vivo expansion of bone marrow stromal cells by platelet-rich plasma: a promising strategy in maxillo-facial surgery. *Int. J. Immunopathol. Pharmacol;* 18:47-53

[13] Meijer, G.J.; de Bruijn, J.D.; Koole, R. & van Blitterswijk, C.A. (2007). Cell-based bone tissue engineering. *PLoS Med*, 4, 260-264.

[14] Caplan, A.I. (2007). Adult mesenchymal stem cells for tissue engineering versus regenerative medicine. *J. Cell Physiol*, 213, 341-347.

[15] Wu, Y.; Chen, L.; Scott, P.G. & Tredget, E.E. (2007). Mesenchymal stem cells enhance wound healing through differentiation and angiogenesis. *Stem Cells*, 25, 2648-2659.

[16] Boyle, W.J.; Simonet, W.S. & Lacey, D.L. (2003) Osteoclast differentiation and activation. *Nature, 423*, 337–342.

[17] Ilan, D.I. & Ladd, A.L. (2003). Bone graft substitutes. *Operat. Tech. Plast. Reconstr. Surg*, 9,151–160.

[18] Damien, C.J. & Parsons, J.R. (1991). Bone grafts and bone graft substitutes: A review of current technology and applications. *J. Appl. Biomater*, 2, 187–208.

[19] Murugan, R. & Ramakrishna, S. (2005) Development of nanocomposites for bone grafting. *Composites Sci. Technol,* 65, 2385–2406.

[20] de Groot, K. (1983). Ceramic of calcium phosphate: Preparation and properties. In: de Groot K (Ed), *Bioceramics of Calcium Phosphate* (pp 100–114). Boca Raton, FL: CRC.

[21] Sato, S.; Koshino, T. & Saito, T. (1998). Osteogenic response of rabbit tibia to hydroxyapatite particle–plaster of Paris mixture. *Biomaterials*, 19, 1895–1900.

[22] Jarcho, M. (1981). Calcium phosphate ceramics as hard tissue prosthetics. *Clin. Orthop. Relat. Res*, 157, 259–278.

[23] Ogiso, M. (1998). Reassessment of long-term use of dense HA as dental implant: Case report. *J. Biomed. Mater Res. B, Appl. Biomater*, 43, 318–320.

[24] Hench, L.L. (1991). Bioceramics: From concept to clinic. *J. Am. Ceram. Soc*, 74, 1487–1510.

[25] Bajpai, P.K. (1992) Ceramics: a novel device for sustained long-term delivery of drugs. In: J.E. Hulbert and S.F. Hulbert Editors, *Bioceramics*. (pp. 87–99). Terre Haute.

[26] Murugan, R. & Ramakrishna, S. (2004). Bioresorbable composite bone paste using polysaccharide based nano hydroxyapatite. *Biomaterials*, 25, 3829–3835.

[27] Komath, M. & Varma, H.K. (2003). Development of a full injectable calcium phosphate cement for orthopedic and dental applications. *Bull. Mater Sci*, 26, 415–422.

[28] Ural, E.; Kesenci, K.; Fambri, L.; Migliaresi, C. & Piskin, E. (2000). Poly(D,Llactide/e-caprolactone)/hydroxyapatite composites. *Biomaterials*, 21, 2147–2154.

[29] Walsh, D.; Furuzono, T. & Tanaka, J. (2001). Preparation of porous composite implant materials by in situ polymerization of porous apatite containing ε-caprolactone or methyl methacrylate. *Biomaterials*, 22, 1205–1211.

[30] Coombes, A.G.A.; Rizzi, S.C.; Williamson, M.; Barralet, J.E.; Downes, S. & Wallace, W.A. (2004). Precipitation casting of polycaprolactone for applications in tissue engineering and drug delivery. *Biomaterials*, 25, 315–325.

[31] Marra, K.G.; Szem, J.W.; Kumta, P.N.; DiMilla, P.A. & Weiss, L.E. (1999). In vitro analysis of biodegradable polymer blend/hydroxyapatite composites for bone tissue engineering. *J. Biomed. Mater Res*, 47, 324–335.

[32] Reis, M. C.; Reis, R. L.; Feijen, M. B.; Feijen, D. W. & Feijen, J. (2003) Development and properties of polycaprolactone/hydroxyapatite composite biomaterials. *J. Mater Sci:Mater M*, 14, 103-107.

[33] Rizzi, S.C.; Heath, D.J.; Coombes, A.G.; Bock, N.; Textor, M. & Downes, S. (2001) Biodegradable polymer/hydroxyapatite composites: Surface analysis and initial attachment of human osteoblasts. *J. Biomed. Mater Res*, 55, 475-486.

[34] Calandrelli, L.; Immirzi, B.; Malinconico, M.; Volpe, M.G.; Oliva, A. & Della Ragione, F. (2000). Preparation and characterisation of composites based on biodegradable polymers for "in vivo" application. *Polymer*, 41, 8027-8033.

[35] Itoh, S.; Kikuchi, M.; Takakuda, K.; Nagaoka, K.; Koyama, Y.; Tanaka, J. & Shinomiya, K. (2002). Implantation study of a novel hydroxyapatite/collagen (HAp/col) composite into weight-bearing sites of dogs. *J. Biomed. Mater Res*, 63, 507–15.

[36] Zhao, F.; Yin, Y.; Lu, W.W.; Leong, J.C.; Zhang, W.; Zhang, J.; Zhang, M. & Yao, K. (2002). Preparation and histological evaluation of biomimetic three-dimensional hydroxyapatite/chitosan-gelatin network composite scaffolds. *Biomaterials, 23,* 3227–34.
[37] Murugan, R. & Panduranga Rao, K. (2002). Biodegradable coralline hydroxyapatite composite gel using natural alginate. *Bioceramics, 15,* 407–10.
[38] Murugan, R. & Panduranga Rao, K. (1998). Synthesis and characterization of bioactive chitosan bonded bone cement for hard tissue replacement. In: Srinivasan KSV (Ed). *Proceedings of the IUPAC Macromolecules.* (pp. 638-641). New Delhi, Allied Publication.
[39] Lakes, R. (1993) Materials with structural hierarchy. *Nature, 361,* 511–515.
[40] Hartgerink, J.D.; Beniash, E. & Stupp, S.I. (2001). Self-assembly and mineralizationùof peptide-amphiphile nanofibers. *Science, 294,* 1684–1688
[41] Suchanek, W. & Yoshimura, M. (1998). Processing and properties of hydroxyapatite-based biomaterials for use as hard tissue replacement implants. *J. Mater Res, 13,* 94–117.
[42] TenHuisen, K.S.; Martin, R.I.; Klimkiewicz, M. & Brown, P.W. (1995). Formation and properties of a synthetic bone composite: hydroxyapatite-collagen. *J Biomed Mater Res, 29,* 803–810.
[43] Webster, T.J.; Siegel, R.W. & Bizios, R. (2000). Enhanced functions of osteoblasts on nanophase ceramics. *Biomaterials, 21,* 1803–1810.
[44] Webster, T.J.; Ergan, C.; Doremus, R.H.; Siegel, R.W. & Bizios, R. (2000). Specific proteins mediate enhanced osteoblast adhesion on nanophase ceramics. *J Biomed Mater Res, 51,* 475–483.
[45] Webster, T.J.; Siegel, R.W. & Bizios, R. (1999). Osteoblast adhesion on nanophase ceramics. *Biomaterials, 20,* 1221–1227.
[46] Rhee, S.H. & Choi, J.Y. (2002). Preparation of a Bioactive Poly(methyl methacrylate)/Silica Nanocomposite. *J. Am. Ceram. Soc, 85,* 1318–1320.
[47] Rhee, S.H. (2003). Effect of calcium salt content in the poly(ε-caprolactone)/silica nanocomposite on the nucleation and growth behavior of apatite layer. *J. Biomed. Mater Res. Part A, 67A,* 1131–1138;
[48] Yoo, J.J. & Rhee, S-H. (2004). Evaluations of bioactivity and mechanical properties of poly (ε-caprolactone)/silica nanocomposite following heat treatment. *J. Biomed. Mater Res. Part A, 68A,* 401–410.
[49] Pecora, G.; Andreana, S.; Margarine, J.E.; Covani, U. & Sottosanti J.S. (1997). Bone regeneration with a calcium sulphate barrier. *Oral. Surg. Oral. Med. Oral. Pathos, 84,* 424-429.

[50] Pecora, G.; De Leonardis, D.; Ibrahim, N.; Bovi, M. & Cornelini, R. (2001). The use of calcium sulphate in the surgical treatment of a "through and trough" periradicular lesion. *Int. Endod. J,* 34, 189-196.
[51] Liu, Q.; de Wijn, J.R.; de Groot, K.; Van Blitterswijk, C.A. (1998). Surface modification of nano-apatite by grafting organic polymer. *Biomaterials,* 19, 1067-1072.
[52] Jagur-Grodzinski, J. (2006). Polymers for tissue engineering, medical devices, and regenerative medicine. Concise general review of recent studies. *Polym. Adv. Technol,* 17, 395–418
[53] Li, W.J. & Tuan, R.S. (2005). Polymeric scaffolds for cartilage tissue engineering. *Macromol. Symp,* 227, 65–75.
[54] Jarcho, M. (1981) Calcium phosphate ceramics as hard tissue prosthetics. *Clin. Orthop. Relat. Res,* 157, 259-278.
[55] Mori, M.; Yamaguchi, M.; *Sumitomo, S. & Takai, Y.* (2004). Hyaluronan-based biomaterials for tissue-engineering. *Acta Histochem. Cytochem,* 37, 1–5.
[56] G.; Tschon, M.; Daly, J. H.; Liggat, J. J.; Fini, M.; Torricelli, P. & Giardino, R. (2004). Natural and synthetic polyesters for musculoskeletal tissue repair: Experimental in vitro and in vivo evaluation. *Int. J. Artificial. Organs,* 27, 796–805.
[57] Bačáková, L.; Filová, E.; Rypáček, F.; Švorčík, V. & Starý, V. (2004). Cell adhesion on artificial materials for tissue engineering. *Physiological Research,* 53, S35–S45.
[58] Li, Z.; Ramay, HR.; Hauch, K.D.; Xiao, D. & Zhang, M. (2005). Chitosan-alginate hybrid scaffold for bone tissue engineering. *Biomaterials,* 26, 3919–3928.
[59] Cowin, S.C.; Vanburskirk, W.C. & Ashaman, R.B. (1987).. In: Skalak, R.; Chien, S. editors, *Handbook of Bioengineering* (p. 97). New York: McGraw Hill.
[60] Sato, T.; Chen, G.; Ushida, T.; Ishii, T.; Ochiai, N.; Tateishi, T. & Tanaka, J. (2004). Evaluation of PLLA-collagen hybrid sponge as a scaffold for cartilage tissue engineering. *Mater Sci. Eng. C,* 24, 365–372.
[61] Schantz, J.T.; Brandwood, A.; Hutmacher, D.W.; Khor, H.L.& Bittner, K. (2005) Osteogenic differentiation of mesenchymal progenitor cells in computer designed fibrin-polymer-ceramic scaffolds manufactured by fused deposition modeling. *J. Mater. Sci-Mater Med,* 16, 807–819.
[62] Shogren, R.L. & Bagley, E.B. (1999). Natural polymer as advanced materials: some research needs and directions. In S.H. Imam, R.V. Greene and B.R. Zaidi (Eds.), *Biopolymers – utilizing nature's, advanced materials,*

ACS symposium series 723 (pp. 2–11). Washington, Oxford University Press.

[63] Kaplan, D.L. (1998). *Biopolymers from renewable resources: Introduction to polymers from renewable resources*. In: Kaplan DL (Ed). Berlin, Germany: Springer Verlag.

[64] Yannas IV. (1996). *Biomaterials science: An introduction to materials in medicine. Natural materials*. In: Ratner BD, HoffmanAS, Schoen FJ, Lemons JE (Eds), California, USA: Academic Press.

[65] Miyamoto, T.; Takahashi, S.; Ito, H.; Inagaki, H. & Noishiki, Y. (1989). Tissue biocompatibility of cellulose and its derivatives. *J. Biomed. Mater Res*, 23, 125-133.

[66] Hayashi, T. (1994). Biodegradable polymers for biomedical uses. *Prog. Polym. Sci*, 19, 663-702.

[67] Ravi Kumar, M.N.V.; Muzzarelli, R.A.A; Muzzarelli, C.; Sashiwa, H. & Domb, A.J. (2005). Chitosan chemistry and pharmaceutical perspectives. *Chem. Rev*, 104, 6017–6083.

[68] Jayakumar, R.; Prabaharan, M.; Reis, R.L. & Mano, J.F. (2005). Graft copolymerized chitosanpresent status and applications. *Carbohydr. Polym*, 62, 142–158.

[69] Bernkop-Schnurch, A.; Hornof, M. & Guggi, D. (2004). Thiolated chitosans. *Eur. J. Pharm. Biopharm*, 57, 9–17.

[70] Ishihara, M.; Ono, K.; Sato, M.; Nakanishi, K.; Saito, Y.; Yra, H.; Matsui, T.; Hattori, H.; Fujita, M.; Kikuchi, M. & Kurita, A. (2001). Acceleration of wound contraction and healing with a photocrosslinkable chitosan hydrogel. *Wound Rep. Reg*, 9, 513-21.

[71] Razania, A. & Healy, K.E. (1999). Biomimetic peptide surfaces that regulate adhesion, spreading , cytoskeletal organization, and mineralization of the matrix deposited by osteoblast-like cells. *Biotechnol. Prog*, 15, 19-32.

[72] Park, Y.J.; Lee, Y.M.; Park, S.N.; Sheen, S.Y.; Chung, C.P. & Lee, S.J. (2000). Platelet derived growth factor releasing chitosan sponge for periodontal bone regeneration. *Biomaterials*, 21, 153-159.

[73] Klokkevold, P.R.; Vandemark, L.; Kenney, E.B.; Bernard, G.W. (1996). Osteogenesis enhanced by chitosan poly(N-acetyl glucosaminoglycan) in vitro. *J. Periodontol*, 67, 1170-175.

[74] Muzzarelli, R.A.; Mattioli-Belmonte, M.; Tietz, C.; Biagini, R.; Ferioli, G.; Brunelli, M.A.; Fini, M.; Giardino, R.; Ilari, P. & Biagini, G. (1994). Stimulatory effect on bone formation exerted by a modified chitosan. *Biomaterials*, 15, 1075-1081.

[75] Chandy, T. & Sharma, C.P. (1993). Chitosan matrix for oral sustained delivery of ampicillin. *Biomaterials*, 14, 939-44.

[76] Hirano, S.; Tsuchida, H.; Nagao, N. (1989). N-acetylation in chitosan and the rate of its enzymatic hydrolysis. *Biomaterials*, 10, 574-576.

[77] Kuen, Y.L.; Wuan, S.H. & Won, H.P. (1995). Blood compatibility and biodegradability of partially N-acylated chitosan derivatives. *Biomaterials*, 16, 1211-216.

[78] Park, Y. J.; Lee, Y. M.; Park, S. N.; Sheen, S. Y.; Chung, C. P. & Lee, S. J. (2000). Platelet derived growth factor releasing chitosan sponge for periodontal bone regeneration. *Biomaterials*, 21, 153-159.

[79] Klokkevold, P. R.; Vandemark, L.; Kenney, E. B. & Bernard, G. W. (1996). Osteogenesis Enhanced by Chitosan in vitro. *J. Periodontol*, 67, 1170-1175.

[80] Gutowska, A.; Jeong, B. & Jasionowski, M. (2001). Injectable gels for tissue engineering. *Anatomical Record*, 263, 342-349.

[81] Malette, W. G.; Quigley, H. & Adickes, E. D. (1986). *Chitosan Effect in Nature and Technology: Chitin in nature and technology.* In: Muzzarelli, R.; Jeuiaux, C.; Gooddy, G. W. (Eds.), New York, Plenum Press.

[82] Somashekar, D. & Joseph, R. (1996). Chitosanase-properties and applications: a review. *Bioresour. Technol*, 55, 35-45.

[83] Murugan, R. & Ramakrishna, S. (2004). Bioresorbable composite bone paste using polysaccharide based nano hydroxyapatite. *Biomaterials*, 25, 3829–3835.

[84] Yang, D.; Jin, Y.; Ma, G.; Chen, X.; Lu, F. & Nie, J. (2008). Fabrication and characterization of chitosan/PVA with hydroxyapatite biocomposite nanoscaffolds. *J. Appl. Polym. Sci*, 110, 3328–3335.

[85] Aiedeh, K. & Taha, M.O. (1999). Synthesis of chitosan succinate and chitosan phthalate and their evaluation as suggested matrices in orally administered, colon-specific drug delivery systems. *Arch. Pharm*, 332, 103–107.

[86] Liu, Y.F.; Huang, K.L.; Peng, D.M.; Ding, P. & Li, G.Y. (2007). Preparation and characterization of glutaraldehyde cross-linked O-carboxymethylchitosan microspheres for controlled delivery of pazufloxacin mesilate. *Int. J. Biol. Macromol*, 41, 87–93.

[87] Wang, X. (1998). Calcium alginate gels: formation and stability in the presence of an inert electrolyte. *Polymer*, 39, 2759-2764.

[88] LeRoux, M.A. (1999). Compressive and shear properties of alginate gel: effects of sodium ions and alginate concentration. *J. Biomed. Mater. Res*, 47, 46-53.

[89] Mumper, R.J. (1994). Calcium alginate beads for the oral delivery of TGF-betal. *J. Control. Release*, 30, 241-251.
[90] Zhang, S. M.; Cui, F. Z.; Liao, S. S.; Zhu, Y. & Han, L. (2003). Synthesis and biocompatibility of porous nano-hydroxyapatite/collagen/alginate composite. *J. Mater Sci: Mater Med*, 14, 641-645.
[91] Parhi, P.; Ramanan, A. & Ray, A.R. (2006). Preparation and characterization of alginate and hydroxyapatite-based biocomposite. *J. Appl. Polym. Sci*, 102, 5162–5165.
[92] Tampieri, A.; Sandri, M.; Landi, E.; Celotti, G.; Roveri, N.; Mattioli-Belmonte, M.; Virgili, L.; Gabbanelli, F. & Biagini, G. (2005). HA/alginate hybrid composites prepared through bio-inspired nucleation *Acta Biomaterialia*, 1, 343-351.
[93] Bottini, M.; Cerignoli, F.; Dawson, M.I.; Magrini, A.; Rosato, N. & Mustelin, T. (2006). Full-Length Single-Walled Carbon Nanotubes Decorated with Streptavidin-Conjugated Quantum Dots as Multivalent Intracellular Fluorescent Nanoprobes. *Biomacromolecules*, 7, 2259-2263.
[94] Bottini, M.; Magrini, A.; Di Venere, A.; Bellucci, S.; Dawson, M.I.; Rosato, N.; Bergamaschi, A. & Mustelin, T. (2006). Synthesis and Characterization of Supramolecular Nanostructures of Carbon Nanotubes and Ruthenium-Complex Luminophores. *J. Nanosci. Nanotechnol*, 6, 1381-1386.
[95] Wang, J.; Zhang, K. & Zhu, Y. (2005). Synthesis of SiO_2-Coated $ZnMnFe_2O_4$ nanospheres with Improved Magnetic Properties. *J. Nanosci. Nanotechnol*, 5, 772-775.
[96] Lin, Y.W.; Liu, C.W. & Chang, H.T. (2006). Synthesis and Properties of Water-Soluble Core–Shell–Shell Silica–CdSe/CdS–Silica Nanoparticles. *J. Nanosci. Nanotechnol*, 6, 1092-1100.
[97] Lin, Y.S.; Tsai, C.P.; Huang, H.Y.; Kuo, C.T.; Hung, Y.; Huang, D.M.; Chen, Y.C. & Mou, C.Y. (2005). Well-Ordered Mesoporous Silica Nanoparticles as Cell Markers. *Chem. Mater*, 17, 4570–4573.
[98] Bharali, D.J.; Klejbor, I.; Stachowiak, E.K.; Dutta, P.; Roy, I.; Kaur, N.; Bergey, E.J.; Prasad, PN. & Stachowiak, K.M. (2005). Organically modified silica nanoparticles: A nonviral vector for *in vivo* gene delivery and expression in the brain. *PNAS*, 102, 11539-11544.
[99] Yang, J.M.; Lu, C.S.; Hsu, Y.G. & Shih, C.H. (1997). Mechanical Properties of Acrylic Bone Cement Containing PMMA–SiO2 Hybrid Sol–Gel Material, *J. Biomed. Mater Res. B, Appl. Biomater*, 38B, 143–54.
[100] Wei, Y. & Jin, D. (1997). A New Class of Organic-Inorganic Hybrid Dental Materials. *Polym. Prepr*, 38, 122–123.

[101] Paul, P.P.; Timmons, S.F.W. & Machowski, J. (1997). Organic-Inorganic Hybrid Dental Restorative Composites. *Polym. Prepr*, 38, 124-125.
[102] Yoo, J.J. & Rhee, S-H. (2004). Evaluations of bioactivity and mechanical properties of poly (ε-caprolactone)/silica nanocomposite following heat treatment. *J. Biomed. Mater Res. Part A,* 68A, 401–410.
[103] Wei, J.; Heo, S. J.; Liu, C.; Kim, D. H.; Kim, S. E.; Hyun, Y. T.; Shin, J.-W. & Shin, J.-W. (2009). Preparation and characterization of bioactive calcium silicate and poly(ε-caprolactone) nanocomposite for bone tissue regeneration. *J. Biomed. Mater Res. Part A,* 90, 702-712.
[104] Xu, T.; Zhang, N; Nichols, H. L.; Shi, D. & Wen, X. (2007). Modification of nanostructured materials for biomedical applications. *Mater. Sci. Eng. C,* 27, 579–594.
[105] Redhead, H.M.; Davis, S.S. & Illum, L. (2001). Drug delivery in poly(lactide-co-glycolide) nanoparticles surface modified with poloxamer 407 and poloxamine 908: in vitro characterisation and in vivo evaluation. *J. Control. Release,* 70, 353-363.
[106] Neal, J.C.; Stolnik, S.; Garnett, M.C.; Davis, S.S. & Illum, L. (1998). Modification of the copolymers poloxamer 407 and poloxamine 908 can affect the physical and biological properties of surface modified nanospheres. *Pharm. Res,* 15, 318-324.
[107] Park, Y.J.; Nah, S.H.; Lee, J.Y.; Jeong, J.M.; Chung, J.K.; Lee, M.C.; Yang, V.C. & Lee, S.J. (2003). Surface-modified poly(lactide-co-glycolide) nanospheres for targeted bone imaging with enhanced labeling and delivery of radioisotope. *J. Biom. Mater Res. Part A* 67A, 751-760.
[108] Hrapovic, S.; Liu, Y.L.; Male, K.B. & Luong, J.H.T. (2004). Electrochemical biosensing platforms using platinum nanoparticles and carbon nanotubes. *Analytical Chemistry,* 76, 1083-1088.
[109] Lin, Y.H.; Lu, F.; Tu, Y. & Ren, Z.F. (2004). Glucose biosensors based on carbon nanotube nanoelectrode ensembles. *Nano Letters,* 4, 191-195.
[110] Artyukhin, A.B.; Bakajin, O.; Stroeve, P. & Noy, A. (2004). Layer-by-layer electrostatic self-assembly of polyelectrolyte nanoshells on individual carbon nanotube templates. *Langmuir,* 20, 1442-1448.
[111] Islam, M.F.; Rojas, E.; Bergey, D.M.; Johnson, A.T. & Yodh, A.G. (2003). High weight fraction surfactant solubilization of single-wall carbon nanotubes in water. *Nano Letters,* 3, 269-273.
[112] Nakashima, N.; Tomonari, Y. & Murakami, H. (2002). Water-soluble single-walled carbon nanotubes via noncovalent sidewall-functionalization with a pyrene-carrying ammonium ion. *Chemistry Letters,* 31, 638-639.

[113] Qhobosheane, M.; Santra, S.; Zhang, P. & Tan, W.H. (2001). Biochemically functionalized silica nanoparticles. *Analyst,* 126, 1274-1278.

[114] Moghimi, S.M.; Hunter, A.C. & Murray, J.C. (2001). Long-Circulating and Target-Specific Nanoparticles: Theory to Practice. *Pharmacol. Rev,* 53, 283-318.

[115] Xu, H.; Yan, F.; Monson, E.E. & Kopelman, R. (2003). Room-temperature preparation and characterization of poly (ethylene glycol)-coated silica nanoparticles for biomedical applications. *J. Biom. Mater Res. Part A,* 66A, 870-879.

[116] Butterworth, M.D.; Illum, L. & Davis, S.S. (2001). Preparation of ultrafine silica- and PEG-coated magnetite particles *Colloids and Surfaces A: Physicochem. Eng. Aspects,* 179, 93-102.

[117] Li, S.; Shah, A.; Hsieh, A. J.; Haghighat, R.; Solomon Praveen, S.; Mukherjee, I.; Wei, E.; Zhang, Z. & Wei, Y. (2007). Characterization of poly(2-hydroxyethyl methacrylate-silica) hybrid materials with different silica contents. *Polymer,* 48, 3982-3989.

[118] Kang Y.-M.; Kim, K.-H.; Seol, Y.-J. & Rhee, S.-H. (2009). Evaluations of osteogenic and osteoconductive properties of a non-woven silica gel fabric made by the electrospinning method. *Acta Biomaterialia,* 5, 462–469.

[119] Xua, H. H. K.; Smith, D. T. & Simon, C. G. (2004). Strong and bioactive composites containing nano-silica-fused whiskers for bone repair. *Biomaterials,* 25, 4615–4626.

[120] Beletskii, B. I.; Shumskii, V. I.; Nikitin, A. A. & Vlasova, E. B. (2000). Biocomposite calcium-phosphate materials used in osteoplastic surgery. *Glass and Ceramics,* 57, 322-325.

[121] Coetzee, A.S. (1980). Regeneration of bone in the presence of calcium sulphate. *Arch. Otolaryngol,* 106, 405-409.

[122] Carinci, F.; Piattelli, A.; Stabellini, G.; Palmieri, A.; Scapoli, L.; Laino, G.; Caputi, S. & Pezzetti, F. (2004). Calcium sulfate: Analysis of MG63 osteoblast-like cell response by means of a microarray technology. *J. Biomed. Mater Res. B,* 71, 260-267.

[123] Walsh, W.R.; Morberg, P.; Yu, Y.; Yang, J.L.; Haggard, W; Sheat, P.C.; Svehla, M. & Bruce, J.M. (2002). Response of a calcium sulphate bone graft substitute in a confined cancellous defect. *Clin. Orthop. Relat. Res ,* 406, 228-236.

[124] Ricci, J.L.; Alexander, H.; Nadkarni, P; Hawkins, M.; Turner, J.; Rosenblum, S.; Brezenoff, L.; De Leonardis, D. & Pecora, G. (2000). *Bone engineering: Biological mechanisms of calcium sulfate replacement by bone.* In: Davies JE, editor. Toronto, Canada: Em Squared Inc.

[125] Doadrio, J.C.; Arcos, D.; Cabanas, M.V. & Vallet-Regi, M. (2004). Calcium sulphate-based cements containing cephalexin. *Biomaterials,* 25, 2629-2635.

[126] La Gatta, A.; De Rosa, A.; Laurienzo, P; Malinconico, M.; De Rosa, M. & Schiraldi, C. (2005). A Novel Injectable Poly(epsilon-caprolactone)/Calcium Sulphate System for Bone Regeneration: Synthesis and Characterization. *Macromol. Biosci,* 5, 1108-1117.

[127] Gomez d'Ayala, G.; De Rosa, A.; Laurienzo, P. & Malinconico, M.. (2007). Development of a new calcium sulphate-based composite using alginate and chemically modified chitosan for bone regeneration. *J. Biomed. Mater Res,* 81A, 811–820.

[128] Sosnik, A. & Cohn, D. (2003). Poly(ethylene glycol)-poly(epsilon-caprolactone) block oligomers as injectable materials. *Polymer,* 44, 7033.-7042.

[129] Kweon, H.Y.; Yoo, M.K.; Park, I.K.; Kim, T.H.; Lee, H.C.; Lee, H.S.; Oh, J.-S.; Akaike, T. & Cho, C.-S. (2003). A novel degradable polycaprolactone networks for tissue engineering *Biomaterials,* 24, 801-808.

[130] Stöber, W.; Fink, A. & Bohn, E. (1968). Controlled growth of monodisperse silica spheres in the micron size range. *J Colloid Interfacial Sci,* 26, 62-69.

[131] Lian, J.B. & Stein, G.S. (1992). Concepts of osteoblast growth and differentiation: basis for modulation of bone cell development and tissue formation. *Crit Rev Oral Biol Med,* 3, 269-305.

[132] Majeska, R.J. & Rodan, G.A. (1982). The effects of 1,25(OH)2D3 on alkaline phosphatase in osteoblastic osteosarcoma cells. *J Biol Chem,* 257, 3362-67.

[133] Harada, S. & Rodan, G.A. (2003). Control of osteoblast function and regulation of bone mass. *Nature,* 423, 349-355.

[134] Lee, N.K., Sowa, H.; Hinoi, E.; Ferron, M.; Ahn, J.D.; Confavreux, C.; Dacquin, R.; Mee, P.J.; McKee, M.D.; Jung, D.Y.; Zhang, Z.; Kim, J.K.; Mauvais-Jarvis, F.; Ducy, P. & Karsenty, G. (2007). Endocrine regulation of energy metabolism by the skeleton. *Cell,* 130, 456-69.

[135] Friedenstein, A.J.; Deriglasova, U.F.; Kulagina, N.N.; Panasuk, A.F.; Rudakowa, S.F.; Luria, E.A. & Ruadkow, I.A. (1974). Precursors for fibroblasts in different populations of hematopoietic cells as detected by the in vitro colony assay method. *Exp. Hematol,* 2, 83-92.

[136] Hou, Q.P.; De Bank, P.A. & Shakesheff, K.M. (2004). Injectable scaffolds for tissue regeneration. *J. Mater Chem,* 14, 1915-1923

[137] Nobile, M.R; Pirozzi, V.; Somma, E.; Gomez d'Ayala, G. & Laurienzo, P. (2008). Development and rheological investigation of novel alginate/N-succinylchitosan hydrogels. *J. Polym. Sci. B*, 46, 1167–1182.

[138] Higgs, PG; Ball, RC. (1990). A "reel-chain" model for the elasticity of biopolymer gels, and its relationship to slip-link treatments of entanglements. In *Physical Networks. Polymers and Gels*, Burchard,W and Ross-Murphy, SB, eds.; New York, NY: Elsevier, pp.185-194.

INDEX

A

acetic acid, 69
acetone, 68
acid, 4, 5, 12, 55, 69
acidic, 54, 55
acidity, 13
ACS, 76
activation, 72
adhesion, 1, 10, 11, 20, 23, 25, 28, 32, 37, 42, 49, 74, 75, 76
adipose, 5
adipose tissue, 5
adsorption, 18
adult, 71
age, 47
agent, 12
agents, 16
agricultural, 14
algae, 15
alkaline phosphatase, 34, 40, 42, 49, 62, 81
allogeneic, 6, 9
allograft, 9
alloys, 24, 26, 28, 36, 44, 45, 46
alternative, 53, 67
amine, 18, 55
amines, 17
amino groups, 17
ammonia, 16

ammonium hydroxide, 69
amorphous, 19
angiogenesis, 72
angiogenic, 7
anhydride ring, 55
animal studies, 7
antibiotics, 48
apatite, 17, 73, 74, 75
apatite layer, 18, 74
application, 4, 6, 13, 54, 73
aqueous solution, 56
aqueous suspension, 17
ARS, 69
artificial bone, 9, 16
astrocytes, 6, 71
atmosphere, 36, 47, 48, 49, 61
attachment, 73
autologous bone, 6
availability, 14

B

barrier, 74
barriers, 42
behavior, 7, 74
binding, 17

biocompatibility, 2, 4, 7, 8, 10, 34, 41, 42, 54, 76, 78
biocompatible, 1, 13, 15, 20
biodegradability, 4, 12, 54, 77
biodegradable, 1, 10, 12, 13, 15, 20, 53, 54, 67, 73
biodegradation, 12, 15
bioinert, 36
biological activity, 11
biomaterials, 12, 73, 74, 75
biomedical applications, 15, 41, 67, 79, 80
biomimetic, 14, 15, 16, 74
biomolecule, 17
biopolymer, 11, 82
biopolymers, 2, 10, 14
bioreactor, 6
biosensors, 79
birth, 27
blends, ix, 2, 20, 54, 61
BMA, 32, 33, 35, 37, 38, 39, 40, 42, 43
body fluid, 17, 19, 54
bonding, 10, 11
bone cement, 10, 17, 74
bone graft, 8, 9, 10, 14, 19, 72, 80
bone growth, 9, 54
bone marrow, ix, 2, 5, 6, 34, 35, 42, 47, 61, 71, 72
bone mass, 81
bovine, 41, 50, 64
brain, 78
buffer, 49, 50

C

calcification, 65
candidates, 1
caprolactone, ix, 2, 20, 42, 73, 74, 79, 81
carbon, 79
carbon nanotubes, 79
carboxylic groups, 58, 60
cardiomyocytes, 6
cartilage, 5, 12, 75
casting, 73
catalyst, 17
cell adhesion, 1
cell culture, 43, 68
cell growth, 37, 62, 63, 67
cell line, 71
cell transplantation, 14
cellulose, 76
cement, 20, 57, 73
ceramics, 9, 11, 12, 72, 74, 75
cerebellum, 71
chemical interaction, 11
chemical properties, 24
chemical reactions, 16
chemical structures, 14
chemicals, 8, 43, 68
chitosan, ix, 2, 14, 15, 21, 54, 55, 56, 57, 58, 59, 60, 67, 68, 74, 76, 77, 81
chloroform, 32
colonization, 38
compatibility, ix, 11, 14, 77
complications, 9
components, 4, 10, 12, 28, 57, 60, 67
composition, 9, 11, 12, 21, 28, 35, 59
concentration, 49, 54, 59, 77
condensation, 55
conjugation, 15, 17
connective tissue, 8, 19
consent, 47
control, 11, 37, 38, 40, 41, 45, 61, 62, 63, 64, 65, 67, 69
cooling, 24, 45
copolymers, 13, 79
costs, 14
coupling, 12
covalent, 18, 26
covalent bond, 26
covering, 28
CPC, 18
CRC, 72
crosslinking, 57
crystalline, 17
crystallites, 11
crystallization, 24
crystals, 59
cultivation, 71
culture, 8, 37, 40, 47, 48, 49, 61, 64, 65, 69
cyclohexane, 32

cytokines, 13, 53, 54
cytometry, 48
cytotoxic, 20
cytotoxicity, 7, 8, 42

D

decomposition, 13
defects, 4, 5, 7, 8, 19
deformation, 26
degradation, 13, 24
degree of crystallinity, 24
Degussa, 43
dehydrogenases, 49
delivery, 16, 73, 77, 78, 79
demineralized, 61
denaturation, 54
density, 36, 48
dentistry, 10
deposition, 10, 14, 34, 39, 75
deposits, 19, 54
derivatives, 14, 37, 38, 40, 41, 76, 77
destruction, 8
dexamethasone, 65, 66, 69
dialysis, 68
differentiated cells, 3, 5
differentiation, 10, 18, 34, 39, 42, 61, 62, 64, 72, 75, 81
diffusion, 8, 71
discontinuity, 60
discs, 36, 37, 38, 48
dispersion, 28
distilled water, 56
distribution, 11
DNA, 17
dogs, 73
donor, 47, 48
doped, 16
drug delivery systems, 77
drugs, 73
DSC, 24, 45

E

ECM, 13
egg, 58
elasticity, 82
electrolyte, 77
electron, 60
electron microscopy, 4
electrospinning, 13, 15, 18, 80
encapsulated, 20, 67
encapsulation, 20
endocrine, 40
endothelial cell, 7
energy, 40, 81
entanglements, 82
environment, 53, 54, 61
enzymatic, 77
enzymes, 17
epoxy, 32
ethylene glycol, 80, 81
exposure, 11
extracellular matrix, 13, 34, 62, 65, 67, 69

F

fabric, 18, 80
failure, 7, 11
feedback, 39
fetal, 47
fibers, 65, 67
fibrin, 75
fibroblasts, 5, 36, 43, 81
fillers, 1, 11, 18
film, 44
flexibility, 4
flow, 48
food, 15
forebrain, 71
formaldehyde, 69
fracture, 46
functionalization, 79
fusion, 24, 25

G

gel, 18, 59, 74, 77, 80
gelatin, 74
gelation, 59
gels, 77, 82
gender, 47
gene, 17, 78
gift, 42, 43
glass transition, 24
glutaraldehyde, 77
glycidilmethacrylate, 26
grafting, 20, 75
grafts, 9, 10, 72
groups, 17, 18, 20, 26, 32, 55, 58, 60
growth factor, 6, 7, 12, 53, 54, 76, 77

H

handling, 10, 20
healing, 6, 76
heart, 71
heat, 74, 79
heating, 24, 45
height, 68
hematopoietic cells, 81
heterogeneous, 10, 11
high temperature, 19
histological, 74
homeostasis, 39
homogeneity, 11
homopolymerization, 26
hormone, 39
host, 10
human, ix, 2, 6, 7, 13, 34, 42, 47, 71, 73
human mesenchymal stem cells, 71
humans, 7
hybrid, 13, 18, 75, 78, 80
hydrogels, 20, 82
hydrolysis, 16, 43, 77
hydrophilicity, 32
hydrophobic interactions, 18
hydrophobicity, 13
hydroxide, 69
hydroxyapatite, 1, 9, 14, 16, 39, 72, 73, 74, 77, 78
hypothesis, 59

I

ice, 49
imaging, 16, 79
immobilization, 17
implants, 17, 19, 74
in situ, 6, 16, 45, 53, 73
in vitro, 7, 8, 15, 34, 42, 61, 71, 75, 76, 77, 79, 81
in vivo, 7, 9, 15, 17, 18, 20, 34, 73, 75, 78, 79
incubation, 8, 34, 49
inert, 16, 77
infections, 4
inflammatory, 10
informed consent, 47
injection, 1, 54, 71
injuries, 4
inorganic filler, 12, 60
insertion, 14
integrity, 20, 67
interactions, 18, 24, 25
interdisciplinary, 3
interface, 11, 18, 20, 41
interfacial adhesion, 1, 23, 25, 28, 42
interphase, 25
intrinsic, 1
ionic, 18
ions, 15, 57, 59, 60, 77
ISO, 7, 8, 34
isolation, 6

K

kinetics, 15

L

labeling, 79
lactic acid, 4, 5
life sciences, 3

limitation, 53
liquid nitrogen, 46
lymphocyte, 72
lysis, 49

M

magnetite, 80
maintenance, 3
mammalian cell, 7
marrow, 5, 14, 71
matrix, 10, 11, 13, 18, 20, 24, 25, 27, 28, 34, 39, 44, 45, 54, 60, 61, 62, 65, 66, 67, 69, 76, 77
measurement, 34
mechanical properties, ix, 2, 9, 12, 17, 18, 20, 27, 41, 58, 74, 79
medicine, 3, 76
melt, 1
mesenchymal progenitor cells, 75
mesenchymal stem cell, ix, 2, 5, 71, 72
mesenchymal stem cells, ix, 2, 5, 71, 72
metabolism, 40, 81
metals, 9
methanol, 68
methyl methacrylate, 73, 74
micelles, 16
microarray technology, 80
microenvironment, 7
microscope, 8, 46
microspheres, 77
migration, 13, 15
mineralization, 34, 39, 62, 65, 66, 69, 76
minerals, 8, 10
mitogenic, 72
mixing, 24, 26, 45
modeling, 75
modified polymers, 56
modulation, 6, 81
modulus, 25, 27, 33, 41, 57
molar ratio, 17, 68
molecular weight, 20, 42, 67, 68
molecules, 3, 6, 12, 16, 18, 54, 59
monoclonal antibodies, 48
monomer, 32

monomers, 18, 32
morphological, 8, 18, 23, 34, 59
morphology, 11, 15, 28, 41, 46, 61, 62, 63
moulding, 68
mouse, 71
multipotent, 48
murine cell, 34
muscle, 6
musculoskeletal, 13, 75

N

nanocomposites, 17, 24, 25, 26, 27, 28, 30, 32, 33, 35, 41, 42, 44, 45, 46, 61, 68, 72
nanocrystals, 16
nanofibers, 13, 74
nanofiller, 28
nanometer, 10, 11
nanoparticles, ix, 1, 11, 16, 17, 18, 20, 23, 24, 25, 26, 27, 34, 43, 46, 78, 79, 80
nanoreactors, 16
nanostructured materials, 79
nanotubes, 79
natural polymers, 1
neonatal, 71
neovascularization, 7
network, 4, 5, 15, 59, 65, 74
neurons, 6, 71
neurosurgery, 10
nitrogen, 46
nodules, 65, 67
nontoxicity, 14
nucleation, 16, 17, 74, 78
nucleophilicity, 55
nutrients, 7

O

oil, 16
oligomers, 81
oligonucleotides, 17
optical, 49
optimization, 12
oral, 77, 78

organ, 3
organic, 1, 10, 11, 12, 13, 18, 75
organism, 11
orthopaedic, 41
osteoblastic cells, 18, 54
osteoblasts, 5, 48, 73, 74
osteocalcin, 34, 40, 42, 48, 49, 50, 62, 64
osteoinductive, 6, 54, 67
osteosarcoma, 81
oxygen, 7

P

particles, 12, 80
penicillin, 46, 47, 48, 61
peptide, 74, 76
periodontal, 76, 77
pharmaceutical, 76
phenol, 49
phenotype, ix, 2, 39, 71
phenotypic, 48
phosphate, 8, 11, 18, 19, 50, 54, 72, 73, 75
physical and mechanical properties, ix, 2
physical properties, 33
physiological, 19, 54
plasma, 6, 72
plastic, 25
plasticity, 6
platelet, 6, 72
platforms, 79
platinum, 79
PLGA, 13
PLLA, 13, 75
PMMA, 78
PMSF, 49
poly(L-lactide), 13
polycondensation, 43
polyester, 20, 25, 41
polymer, 4, 11, 14, 20, 24, 27, 28, 45, 54, 55, 59, 67, 68, 73, 75
polymer chains, 60
polymer matrix, 20, 24, 27, 28, 45, 54, 59
polymer systems, 20
polymer-based, 67
polymerization, 73

polymers, ix, 1, 9, 10, 12, 13, 15, 20, 21, 56, 59, 73, 76
polypeptide, 50
polysaccharide, 15, 55, 58, 73, 77
polystyrene, 36, 47
poor, 15
population, 6
pore, 4, 5, 15
pores, 4
porous, 4, 13, 19, 53, 73, 78
powder, 19, 57, 68
power, 58
precipitation, 16, 32, 54, 55
precursor cells, 5
pressure, 44, 68
pristine, 55, 56
production, 19
progenitors, 8
proliferation, 10, 13, 34, 37, 49, 62, 65, 72
prosthetics, 72, 75
protein, 39, 49, 50
proteins, 17, 54, 74
protocol, 68
PVA, 77
pyrene, 79

R

radioisotope, 79
range, 37, 56, 81
reactive groups, 32
reactivity, 17
reagent, 18, 43
reconstruction, 12
reconstructive surgery, 1, 9
regenerate, 10
regeneration, ix, 1, 6, 8, 12, 13, 14, 15, 17, 18, 20, 54, 56, 60, 74, 76, 77, 79, 81
regenerative medicine, 3, 72, 75
regular, 38
regulation, 40, 81
reinforcement, 1, 25, 57, 67
relationship, 82
reliability, 47
remodeling, 8

Index

renewable resource, 76
repair, 3, 13, 15, 54, 75, 80
reservoir, 8
resin, 17, 18
resources, 76
rigidity, 41
risk, 54
room temperature, 46, 61, 68, 69

S

salt, 54, 74
salts, 11, 17, 19
sample, 36, 45, 47
sand, 16
scaffolds, 6, 13, 15, 42, 53, 54, 67, 74, 75, 81
scanning electron microscopy, 4
secrete, 7
seeding, 39
self-assembly, 79
self-renewal, 5
SEM micrographs, 30, 32
series, 48, 76
serum, 41, 47, 50, 64
serum albumin, 41, 50, 64
shape, 14, 23, 53, 57, 62, 67
shear, 77
short period, 10
sign, 11
signals, 4, 6
signs, 8
silane, 18
silicate, 19, 79
silicon, 36
simulated body fluid, 17
single-wall carbon nanotubes, 79
sintering, 19
sites, 73
skeleton, 8, 39, 81
skin, 12
SNP, 16
sodium, 47, 48, 77
solubility, 14, 15, 56
solvents, 68
specific surface, 48

speed, 27, 45, 46, 68
spheres, 81
spindle, 47
stability, 14, 24, 77
standard deviation, 50
standards, 34
STD, 57
stem cells, 3, 5, 14, 53, 71, 72
strategies, 12
strength, 4, 11, 19, 57
stress, 25, 27
stroma, 6
stromal, 5, 34, 35, 40, 42, 48, 61, 64, 71, 72
stromal cells, 5, 34, 35, 40, 42, 48, 64, 71, 72
structural defect, 27
structural defects, 27
substitutes, 3, 14, 20, 72
sulfate, 80
supernatant, 47, 69
supplements, 6
supply, 7, 9
surface area, 16
surface modification, 12
surface properties, 12
surfactant, 17, 79
surgery, 10, 41, 72, 80
surgical, 53, 75
swelling, 14
synergistic, 21, 58, 59
synergistic effect, 21, 58, 59
synthesis, 19, 40, 41, 50, 64
synthetic bone, 9, 74
synthetic polymers, 12, 13, 14
systems, ix, 2, 20, 26, 28, 53, 77

T

TCP, 11, 19
technology, 72, 77
TEM, 23, 24, 46
temperature, 15, 17, 19, 44, 45, 68, 80
temporal, 39
tendon, 6
tensile, 25, 27, 32
TEOS, 43

tetraethoxysilane, 43
TGF, 78
thermal analysis, 26, 45
thermal stability, 24
three-dimensional, 74
tibia, 72
time, 17, 19, 44, 48, 53, 54, 57
tissue engineering, 3, 5, 6, 7, 12, 13, 15, 16, 42, 54, 67, 72, 73, 75, 77, 81
tissue-engineering, 75
toxic, 10, 15
toxicity, 8, 35
trabecular bone, 19
traction, 46
transfer, 9
transformation, 57
transition, 24
transition temperature, 24
Transmission Electron Microscopy, 23
transplantation, 14, 71
tumors, 4

U

uniform, 11, 13

V

values, 33, 37, 38, 40, 41, 50, 56, 62, 64
variability, 47
variation, 14, 24
vascularization, 7
vector, 17, 78
vehicles, 16
versatility, 14

W

water, 13, 14, 15, 16, 19, 43, 46, 55, 56, 67, 79
water-soluble, 55
wells, 49
workability, 15
wound healing, 15, 72